Palliative Care within Mental Health

CARE AND PRACTICE

Edited by

DAVID B COOPER

Sigma Theta Tau International: The Honor Society of Nursing Award
Nursing Council on Alcohol: Outstanding Contribution to Nursing Award
Editor-in-Chief, *Mental Health and Substance Use*
Author/Writer/Editor

and

JO COOPER

Macmillan Clinical Nurse Specialist in Palliative Care (Retired)
Award in Specialist Practice
Author/Editor

Radcliffe Publishing
London • New York

Radcliffe Publishing Ltd
St Mark's House
Shepherdess Walk
London N1 7BQ
United Kingdom

www.radcliffehealth.com

British Library Cataloguing in Publication Data

A catalogue record for this book is available from the British Library.

ISBN-13: 978 184619 891 5

The paper used for the text pages of this book
is FSC® certified. FSC (The Forest Stewardship
Council®) is an international network to promote
responsible management of the world's forests.

Typeset by Darkriver Design, Auckland, New Zealand
Manufacturing managed by 21six

Contents

Preface

The book is not just about caring for the dying within mental health but about applying the quality care and practice of palliative care within mental health practice. The book focuses on intervention, treatment, care and practice and the similarities in practice between palliative care and mental health.

The common ground is an excellent foundation in care and practice for integrating palliative care, now recognised as best-practice end-of-life care, into mental health care, practice and service delivery. In short, the shared practice values and vision between these two disciplines provide for a starting point for integrated intervention, treatment, care and practice using best practices from palliative care and mental health.

The book came into being when we (the editors) were talking and the discussion led on to the need for more information and direction when it comes to humanness and the issue of palliative care within mental health practice. Whilst it could be assumed that mental health has a lot to offer palliative care, we both felt that palliative care could offer more to mental health practice in that it is a neglected area. There is little or no literature related to palliative care within mental health practice, and that which does exist relates to care of the dying in terms of cancer.

What struck us was that several chapters covered within the *Mental Health–Substance Use* series of books (*see* Other books by the editors, p. xviii) could equally apply to palliative care within mental health care and practice. In the time it took us to drink our coffee we had developed a contents list! As the title *Palliative Care within Mental Health: care and practice* suggests, the whole approach would be on the human aspects of care and practice.

Is there a place for palliative care within mental health? At the mention of palliative care, there is a general assumption that:
1   the person has a cancer diagnosis and
2   the person is dying.

However, this is not the true meaning of palliation. A simple understanding might be that if one has ill-health that is serious and enduring (even with periods of respite) then that person needs careful and continuous symptom management together with skilled emotional support so that she or he can achieve the best quality of life with managed symptom control as effectively as possible – that is palliative care.

We have combined our different skills (Jo – palliative care; David – mental health) to edit this book and a highly qualified team were invited to contribute. We hope we have edited a thought-provoking and informative text on *palliative care within mental health care and practice.*

David B Cooper and Jo Cooper
June 2014

About the editors

David B Cooper
Sigma Theta Tau International: Honor Society of Nursing Award
Nursing Council on Alcohol: Outstanding Contribution to Nursing Award
Editor-in-Chief: *Mental Health and Substance Use*
Author/Writer/Editor
Horsham, West Sussex, England

David has specialised in mental health and substance use for over 34 years. He has worked as a practitioner, manager, researcher, author, lecturer and consultant. He has served as editor, or editor-in-chief, of several journals, and is currently editor-in-chief of *Mental Health and Substance Use*. He has published widely and is 'credited with enhancing the understanding and development of community detoxification for people experiencing alcohol withdrawal' (Nursing Council on Alcohol; Sigma Theta Tau International citations). Seminal work includes *Alcohol Home Detoxification and Assessment* and *Alcohol Use*, both published by Radcliffe Publishing, Oxford. David (2011) edited a series of six textbooks with the series title of *Mental Health–Substance Use*.

Jo Cooper
Macmillan Clinical Nurse Specialist in Palliative Care (retired)
Author/Editor
Horsham, West Sussex, England

Jo spent 16 years in specialist palliative care, initially working in a hospice inpatient unit, then 12 years as a Macmillan Clinical Nurse Specialist in Palliative Care. She gained a Diploma in Oncology at Addenbrooke's Hospital, Cambridge, and a BSc (Hons) in Palliative Nursing at The Royal Marsden, London, and an Award in Specialist Practice. Jo edited *Stepping into Palliative Care* (2000) and the 2nd edition, *Stepping into Palliative Care 1: relationships and responses* (2006) and *Stepping into Palliative Care 2: care and practice* (2006), both published by Radcliffe Publishing. Jo has been involved in teaching for many years and her specialist subjects include management of complex pain and symptoms, terminal agitation, communication at the end-of-life, therapeutic relationships and breaking bad news.

The editors welcome approaches and feedback, positive and/or negative.

List of contributors

CHAPTER 1
Jo Cooper and David B Cooper
See About the editors, p. vii.

CHAPTER 2
David B Cooper
See About the editors, p. vii.

CHAPTER 3
Professor Cynthia MA Geppert
Chief, Consultation Psychiatry and Ethics, New Mexico Veterans Affairs Health Care System
Professor, Department of Psychiatry and Director of Ethics and Professionalism Education, University of New Mexico School of Medicine
Albuquerque, New Mexico, USA

Cynthia is Chief of Consultation Psychiatry and Ethics and Integrated Ethics Program Officer at the New Mexico Veterans Affairs Health Care System. She is also Associate Professor in the Department of Psychiatry and Director of Ethics Education at the University of New Mexico School of Medicine. Cynthia is board certified in general psychiatry, psychosomatic medicine, hospice and palliative medicine, and addiction medicine and holds credentials in pain management. Cynthia is a fellowship and graduate-trained bioethicist with a specialty in religious and clinical ethics and the ethics of addiction.

CHAPTER 4
Professor Geraldine S Pearson
Child and Adolescent Psychiatry, University of Connecticut School of Medicine
Farmington, Connecticut, USA

Geraldine is an Associate Professor at the University of Connecticut School of Medicine. She is the director of the HomeCare Program, a short-term psychiatric medication management programme for adolescents involved in juvenile justice.

Her education is from the University of Cincinnati (BSN & MSN) and University of Connecticut (PhD). She is the editor of *Perspectives in Psychiatric Nursing* and an elected member of the Committee on Publication Ethics (COPE).

CHAPTER 5

Professor Robin Davidson
Consultant Clinical Psychologist
Department of Health, Isle of Man
Belfast, Northern Ireland

Robin is a Consultant Clinical Psychologist and has published widely in addictions, health psychology and psycho-oncology. He left the Leeds Addiction Unit in 1984 to become Head of Clinical Psychology Services for the Northern Health and Social Board and then in 1997 became director of psychological services in the Belfast City Hospital. It was when with the BCH that he developed and managed the Macmillan Support and Information Centre. He has honorary appointments with Queen's University Belfast, the University of Ulster and London South Bank University. He left the NHS several years ago and is contracted to the Isle of Man Health Psycho-oncology service. He is currently Co-chair of GAIN (the NI equivalent of NICE) and Chair of Alcohol Research UK, formerly AERC.

Dr Tracy Anderson
Southern Area Hospice Services
Newry, Northern Ireland

Tracy is a Consultant in Palliative Medicine working in the Southern Trust, Northern Ireland. She works in two acute hospitals, a specialist palliative care unit and additionally has some input into the care of patients in the community. Her main role, as part of a multidisciplinary team, is to provide symptom relief and psychological support for patients with advanced progressive, incurable illness. She has a particular interest in the use of cognitive behavioural therapy (CBT) and has published on cognitive behavioural therapy techniques for anxiety and depression tailored specifically for palliative care. She delivers training workshops on psychological interventions in end-of-life care.

CHAPTER 6

Jo Cooper
See About the editors, p. vii.

CHAPTER 7

Dr John R Ashcroft
Consultant Psychiatrist, The Brooker Centre, Halton General Hospital
Runcorn, England

John is currently employed as a Locum Consultant Psychiatrist at 5 Boroughs Partnership NHS Foundation Trust. He studied Medicine at Imperial College, London and qualified in 2000. He became a member of the Royal College of Psychiatrists in 2006. His has a special interest in neuropsychiatry and addiction. In 2008 he was awarded a Postgraduate Diploma in Clinical Neuropsychiatry with Merit from the University of Birmingham. John is on the international advisory board for the journal *Mental Health and Substance Use*. He also undertakes manuscript and book reviews.

CHAPTER 8

Dr Peter Athanasos
Adjunct Senior Lecturer, Discipline of Psychiatry, Flinders University
Adelaide, Australia

Peter is a mental health nurse and researcher working in Adelaide, Australia. His PhD was in the pharmacology of addictions. Peter's main area of research interest is the effect of substance use on co-existing disorders such as mental illness, pain and other pathophysiology. He has published more than 40 articles, chapters and articles in these areas. He is currently National Secretary and South Australian Representative for the Australasian Professional Society on Alcohol and other Drugs (APSAD).

Trevor W Mitten
Higher Education Success Tutor in Palliative Care, Truro and Penwith College
Truro, England

Trevor has worked in palliative care for over 18 years. After five years at the newly built Exeter Hospice, he moved to North Devon Hospice and spent 11 years as a hospice community charge nurse and clinical nurse specialist in palliative care. Following two and a half years as a Macmillan Nurse, Trevor worked as a Gold Standards co-ordinator in the independent sector. Trevor holds a bachelor's degree with honours in health studies and a postgraduate certificate in enhanced palliative care. Previous publications include an article on syringe drivers, and book chapters on pain control, syringe drivers and pain management. Trevor combines his nursing role with being a higher education tutor in palliative care short courses, leading to a Certificate of Professional Development at Truro and Penwith College.

Dr Rose Neild
Adjunct Senior Lecturer, School of Public Health, Flinders University
Affiliated Senior Lecturer, School of Health Sciences, University of Adelaide
Senior Consultant, Northern Drug and Alcohol Services SA
Elizabeth, South Australia, Australia

Rose works as an Addiction Medicine Consultant for Drug and Alcohol Services South Australia. She also holds an adjunct senior lecturer position at the School of Public Health, Flinders University of South Australia and an affiliate senior lecturer position in the Discipline of Pharmacology, University of Adelaide. She is the current President of the Australasian Professional Society on Alcohol and other Drugs (APSAD), a member of the APSAD Scientific Program Committee and a reviewer for the peer-reviewed *Medical Journal of Australia*. She is a foundation fellow of the Royal Australasian College of Physician's Chapter of Addiction Medicine. Rose is a current student in the Master of Medicine (pain management) course at Sydney University and is also completing her Doctor of Public Health at Flinders University. Rose has a particular interest in working with women with substance use disorders, especially those who are pregnant or parenting as well as those with pain issues attending drug and alcohol services or within broader healthcare environments. Other interest areas include physical and psychiatric comorbidities with dependence in both clinical and public health arenas. Rose is widely published in the area of trauma, mental health and substance use, and more recently the impact of substance use on parenting.

Professor Charlotte de Crespigny
Professor of Drug and Alcohol Nursing, University of Adelaide
Adelaide, South Australia, Australia

Charlotte is a registered nurse who has been working in the drug and alcohol field as a clinician, educator and researcher since 1988. Charlotte's current research interests include: systems of care; alcohol, drug and mental health comorbidity; co-ordinated Aboriginal mental health care; Aboriginal people's use of over-the-counter analgesics; women, alcohol and licensed premises; social drinking in context; and heatwave and the impact on vulnerable people with mental health and substance use conditions. Charlotte works in partnership with other researchers, service leaders and practitioners from varying health fields including general healthcare, mental health, alcohol and other drugs, public health and health economics, and Aboriginal health. She is committed to translating research findings into everyday healthcare, including clinical practice, health promotion and community and professional education – in both government and non-government sectors. Charlotte has many journal publications, best practice guidelines and chapters in texts.

Dr Lynette Cusack
Senior Lecturer, University of Adelaide School of Nursing
Adelaide, South Australia, Australia

Lynette holds a senior lecturer position with the University of Adelaide School of Nursing. Lynette previously worked in the alcohol and other drugs field for over 14 years in an executive role with the Drug and Alcohol Services SA (DASSA), which is a state government organisation.

CHAPTER 9

Philip James
Clinical Nurse Specialist in Adolescent Substance Misuse, Youth Drug and Alcohol
Service, Health Service Executive
Tallaght, Ireland

Philip trained as a psychiatric nurse in Dublin 1999 and was appointed as the first
Clinical Nurse Specialist in Adolescent Substance Misuse in 2006. Since then he has
worked in the HSE's Youth Drug and Alcohol (YoDA) Service full-time. He completed
a master's degree in 2005 and is a qualified cognitive behavioural therapist. In addition
to his clinical work he has been involved in a number of research projects and publications. He has published various research articles and is co-author of *Adolescents and
Substance Use: the handbook for professionals working with young people*, which was
published by Radcliffe Publishing in 2013. He is a reviewer for three international academic journals and is on the International Advisory Committee of the journal *Mental
Health and Substance Use*. He provides lectures on a variety of addiction and mental
health-related topics at a number of colleges, including University College Dublin,
Trinity College Dublin, University of Limerick and the Irish College of Humanities
and Applied Sciences.

CHAPTER 10

Dr Alyna Turner
Senior Clinician, School of Medicine and Public Health, University of Newcastle
Callaghan, New South Wales, Australia

Alyna is a clinical psychologist who has practiced in liaison psychiatry, psychiatric
rehabilitation and community chronic illness services over the last 13 years. She is currently Senior Clinician at the University of Newcastle and Research Fellow at Deakin
University, Australia. She has contributed to trials in evaluating integrated psychological
treatment for mental health-substance use problems and research into assessment and
treatment of mental health problems in people with chronic physical illness.

Dr Stephanie Oak
Head of Department, Liaison Psychiatry, John Hunter Hospital
New Lambton Heights, New South Wales, Australia

Stephanie is a senior psychiatrist and pain medicine physician. She is currently Head
of Department of the Liaison Psychiatry Unit at John Hunter Hospital, Newcastle,
Australia and is a conjoint senior lecturer at the School of Medicine and Public Health,
Faculty of Health, University of Newcastle.

Professor Brian Kelly
School of Medicine and Public Health, University of Newcastle
Callaghan, New South Wales, Australia

Brian is Professor of Psychiatry, School of Medicine and Public Health, Faculty of Health, University of Newcastle. He has a long-standing clinical and research interest in Consultation-Liaison Psychiatry, focusing on psycho-oncology and palliative care and public health aspects of mental illness, including rural mental health.

Professor Amanda L Baker
NHMRC Senior Research Fellow, School of Medicine and Public Health, University of Newcastle
Callaghan, New South Wales, Australia

Amanda is a National Health and Medical Research Council (NHMRC) Senior Research Fellow at the University of Newcastle. She is a senior clinical psychologist who has practised in the United Kingdom and Australia. Her research focuses on the challenging area of the psychological treatment of comorbidity (mental health–substance use problems). She has led numerous trials funded by competitive national grants investigating integrated psychological treatments for these problems and published widely in the field.

CHAPTER 11
Professor Joyce Simard
Adjunct Associate Professor, University of Western Sydney
Private Geriatric Consultant, Land O Lakes
Florida, USA

Joyce is an Adjunct Associate Professor, School of Nursing, University of Western Sydney, Australia and a private geriatric consultant residing in Land O Lakes, Florida and Prague in the Czech Republic. She has been involved in long-term care for over 35 years, serving as Alzheimer's specialist for many healthcare companies, providing services in skilled nursing homes, assisted living communities and hospice organisations. Joyce has written numerous articles and chapters in healthcare books and has authored *The End-of-Life Namaste Care Program for People with Dementia*, now in its second edition.

CHAPTER 12
Dr Kay de Vries
Head of School, Graduate School of Nursing, Midwifery and Health, Victoria University, Wellington
Wellington, New Zealand

Kay is Head of School (Acting) and Director of Research at the Graduate School of Nursing, Midwifery and Health, Victoria University of Wellington, New Zealand. Her research, education and clinical interests are related to all areas of end-of-life care, bereavement, old age and dementia within hospital, the community and care home environments. Her research expertise covers the full range of qualitative methodology and methods. Present research activities range from intensive care nurses' experiences of, and attitudes towards, end-of-life care; palliative care nurse prescribing; bereavement experiences of caregivers of people with dementia; dementia care in acute hospitals; chronic pain in emergency departments; and quality of life in care home facilities. Her doctoral research was focused on the subject of Creutzfeldt–Jakob disease. She holds two affiliate positions, one with the University of Washington, Seattle, USA and the other with the Association for Dementia Studies, University of Worcester, Worcester, UK.

CHAPTER 13
Dr David Ian Jeffrey
Honorary Senior Lecturer in Palliative Care, University of Edinburgh
Headington, Oxford, England

David is an Honorary Lecturer in Palliative Medicine in the University of Edinburgh. Currently he is researching the development of empathy in medical students. David was a general practitioner in Evesham for 20 years, and then became a consultant in palliative medicine in the 3 Counties Cancer Centre, Cheltenham. He was a past Chair of the Ethics Committee of the Association of Palliative Medicine. Latterly, he was Academic Mentor in Dundee Medical School for three years. His books include; *Enhancing Compassion in End-of-Life Care Through Drama: The Silent Treatment* (co-authored with Ewan Jeffrey), *Against Physician Assisted Suicide: a palliative care perspective* and *Patient-Centred Ethics and Communication at the End-of-Life*. David lives with his wife Pru in Oxford and Edinburgh.

CHAPTER 14
Dr Rose Neild
See 'Chapter 8', pp. x–xi.

Dr Peter Athanasos
See 'Chapter 8', p. x.

CHAPTER 15 David B Cooper
See About the editors, p. vii.

Jo Cooper
See About the editors, p. vii.

Terminology

Whenever possible, the following terminology has been applied. However, in certain instances, when referencing a study and/or specific work, when an author has made a specific request, or for the purpose of additional clarity, it has been necessary to deviate from this applied 'norm'.

PROBLEM(S), CONCERNS AND DILEMMAS OR DISORDERS

The terms *problem(s)*, *concerns and dilemmas* and *disorders* can be used interchangeably, as stated by the author's preference. However, where possible, the term 'problem(s)' or 'concerns and dilemmas' has been adopted as the preferred choice.

INDIVIDUAL, PERSON, PEOPLE

There seems to be a need to label the individual – as a form of recognition. Sometimes the label becomes more than the person! 'Alan is schizophrenic' – thus it is Alan, rather than an illness that Alan lives with. We refer to patients, clients, service users, customers, consumers and so on. Yet we feel affronted when we are addressed as anything other than what we are – individuals! We need to be mindful that every person we see during our professional day is an individual – unique. Symptoms are in many ways similar (e.g. delusions, hallucinations), some interventions and treatments are similar (e.g. specific drugs, psychotherapy techniques), but people are not. Alan may experience an illness labelled schizophrenia, and so may John, Beth and Mary, and you or I. However, each will have his or her own unique experiences – and life. None will be the same. To keep this constantly in the mind of the reader, throughout the book we shall refer to the *individual*, *person* or *people* – just like us, but different to us by their uniqueness.

PROFESSIONAL

In the eyes of the individual, we are all professionals, whether students, nurses, doctors, social workers, researchers, clinicians, educationalists, managers, service developers, religious ministers and so on. However, the level of expertise may vary from one professional to another. We are also individuals. There is a need to distinguish between the person experiencing a mental health problem and the person interacting professionally (at whatever level) with that individual. To acknowledge and to differentiate between those who experience – in this context – and those who intervene, we have adopted the term *professional*. It is indicative that we have had, or are receiving, education and training specifically to help us meet the needs of the individual. We may or may not have experienced palliative care and or mental health problems but we have some knowledge that may help the individual – an expertise to be shared. We have a specific knowledge that, hopefully, we wish to use to offer effective intervention and treatment to another human being. It is the need to make a clear differential, and for that purpose only, that forces the use of 'professional' over 'individual' to describe our role – our input into another person's life.

Cautionary note

Wisdom and compassion should become the dominating influences that guide our thoughts, our words, and our actions.[1]

Never presume that what you say is understood. It is essential to check understanding, and what is expected of the individual and/or family, with each person. Each person needs to know what he or she can expect from you, and other professionals involved in her or his care, at each meeting. Jargon is a professional language that excludes the individual and family. Never use it in conversation with the individual, unless requested to do so; it is easily misunderstood.

Remember, we all, as individuals, deal with life differently. It does not matter how many years we have spent studying human behaviour, listening and treating the individual and family. We may have spent many hours exploring with the individual his or her anxieties, fears, doubts, concerns and dilemmas, and the ill-health experience. Yet we do not know what that person really feels, how she or he sees life and ill-health. We may have lived similar lives, experienced the same ill-health, but the individual will always be unique, each different from us, each independent of our thoughts, feelings, words, deeds and symptoms, each with an individual experience.

REFERENCE

1 Matthieu Ricard. As cited in: Föllmi D, Föllmi O. *Buddhist Offerings 365 Days.* London: Thames and Hudson; 2003. p. 30 November.

Other books by the editors

Cooper DB. *Alcohol Home Detoxification and Assessment*. Oxford/New York: Radcliffe Medical Press; 1994. Reprinted 1996.

Cooper DB, editor. *Alcohol Use*. Oxford/New York: Radcliffe Medical Press; 2000. Reprinted 2008.

Cooper DB, editor. *Introduction to Mental Health–Substance Use*. London: Radcliffe Publishing; 2010.

Cooper DB, editor. *Developing Services in Mental Health–Substance Use*. London: Radcliffe Publishing; 2010.

Cooper DB, editor. *Intervention in Mental Health–Substance Use*. London: Radcliffe Publishing; 2011.

Cooper DB, editor. *Responding in Mental Health–Substance Use*. London: Radcliffe Publishing; 2011.

Cooper DB, editor. *Care in Mental Health–Substance Use*. London: Radcliffe Publishing; 2011.

Cooper DB, editor. *Practice in Mental Health–Substance Use*. London: Radcliffe Publishing; 2011.

Cooper J, editor. *Stepping into Palliative Care 1: relationships and responses*. 2nd ed. Oxford/New York: Radcliffe Publishing; 2006.

Cooper J, editor. *Stepping into Palliative Care 2: care and practice*. 2nd ed. Oxford/New York: Radcliffe Publishing; 2006.

Cooper DB, Cooper J, editors. *Palliative Care within Mental Health: principles and philosophy*. London/New York: Radcliffe Publishing; 2012.

Cooper DB, Cooper J, editors. *Palliative Care within Mental Health: care and practice*. London/New York: Radcliffe Publishing; 2014.

Acknowledgements

We are grateful to all the contributors for having the faith in us to produce a valued text and we thank them for their hard work, support and encouragement. We hope that faith proves justified. Thank you to those who have commented along the way, and whose patience has been outstanding.

Many people have helped us along our career paths and life – too many to name individually. Most do not even know what impact they have had on us. Most were individuals who touched our professional lives and who contributed most to our knowledge and understanding, leading us to appreciate the importance of compassion in care ... and our effort to move towards this in practice and life.

To Gillian Nineham of Radcliffe Publishing, our sincere thanks. Gillian had faith in this project from the outset and in our ability to deliver. Her patience is immeasurable and, for that, we are grateful. Thank you also for putting up with our too numerous questions and guiding us through the process of publication! Thank you to Jamie Etherington, Production Development Manager, and Jessica Turner and Alice French of the book marketing department, all competent people who make our work look good. Thanks also to Vivianne Douglas, Project Manager, and Richard Walshe (Copy Editor), and the production team at Darkriver Design, for bringing this book to publication and the many others who are nameless as we write but without whom this book would never come to print; each has his or her stamp on any successes of this book.

Our sincere thanks to our family, friends, and colleagues along our career paths: those who have touched our life in a positive way – and a minority, in a negative way (for we can learn from the negative to ensure we do better for others).

A final heartfelt statement: any errors, omissions, inaccuracies, or deficiencies within these pages are our sole responsibility.

Dedication

This book is dedicated to all those people and their families that we have been privileged to care for. It is they who taught both of us the meaning and the value of compassion, respect and dignity and the life-sustaining importance of hope. It is they who demonstrated to us that the human side of our nature is meaningful and significant in our efforts to care. To them … Thank You.

A special heartfelt dedication must be given to Gillian Nineham, who is not only the person who had faith in us when we met on all the occasions we have written books (since 1994) but who has become a friend and advisor. We are eternally grateful for her guidance and caring, compassionate ways.

Finally, a dedication to five people without whose knowledge of life, love, support and dedication to their children this book would never have been:

Albert (Ted) Edwin Harvey
Emily Harvey
Rose Harvey
Charles (Charlie) Denis Cooper
Joyce Cooper

Never forgotten, may you all rest in peace.

CHAPTER 1

Palliative care within mental health: the need

Jo Cooper, David B Cooper

Perhaps our human purpose is no more or less than that of providing warmth, companionship and acceptance of our fellow women and men, rather than trying to fix them.[1]

INTRODUCTION

This book is about care, practice, intervention and palliative treatment within mental health services. This includes:

➤ person-centred practice
➤ relationship-based connectedness
➤ care and practice
➤ cultural dilemmas
➤ ethical dilemmas
➤ a belief in compassion, respect and dignity in care and practice
➤ respect for autonomy and choice
➤ quality of life issues
➤ the family as the unit of care
➤ the need for democratic and intra-/inter-disciplinary team work.

Palliative Care within Mental Health: care and practice offers an in-depth text to enhance the concepts offered in the first book *Palliative Care within Mental Health: principles and philosophy*. This edition is about the care and practice skills needed for us to be competent to address intervention and treatment in our work environment. Each chapter develops a theoretical and practical framework, and broadens to include application in care practice. Throughout, we adopt a person-centred approach. Both books anticipate that the reader will be able to follow the reasoning for palliative care, within her or his practice, from concept to application.

In this book we develop further the 'What, When, Where and Why'. Overriding to the text is the 'How' in care and practice. Consequently, each chapter moves from informing to implementation – the 'how to'. The aim is to improve, above all else, the relationships, responses, compassion, care and practice necessary to be an effective professional in offering interventions and treatment for those experiencing mental health problems. The emphasis throughout is on the individual *and* the family, compassion and the appreciation of the stigma such problems bring to the individual.

For the individual and family experiencing serious and enduring mental health, life presents many problems. The needs are complex and all-encompassing. For the professional, educator, researcher, manager and service providers/developers, this presents multifaceted challenges. To successfully, and innovatively, deliver interventions, treatment, care and practice responses and comprehensive services, professionals need to continually explore, and update knowledge and skills. *Palliative Care within Mental Health: care and practice* provides discussion and dissemination around the subject of palliative care within mental health. The book does not separate or address 'mental health' or 'palliative care' as individual subjects. Such concerns relate not only to the individual and family but also to the future direction of care, practice, interventions and treatment. Whilst presenting a balanced view of what is best practice today, we aim to challenge concepts and stimulate debate, exploring all aspects of the development of palliative care and practice within mental health and develop appropriate responses incorporating research-led best practice.

WHAT IS PALLIATIVE CARE?

> You matter because you are you. You matter to the last moment of your life, and we will do all we can to help you not only to die peacefully, but also to live until you die.[2]

Palliative care is widely accepted as best practice end-of-life care and is concerned with promoting and maintaining the best possible quality of life. Connecting with the person is the central focus in both palliative care and mental health disciplines. The World Health Organization defines palliative care as:

> an approach that improves the quality of life of patients and their families facing the problems associated with life-threatening illness, through the *prevention and relief of suffering* by means of early identification and impeccable assessment and treatment of pain and other problems, physical, psychosocial and spiritual. Affirms life and regards dying as a normal process that:
> - provides relief from pain and other symptoms
> - intends neither to hasten nor postpone death
> - integrates psychological and spiritual aspects of care
> - offers a support system to help patients to live as actively as possible until death

- offers a support system to help the family cope during the patient's [person's] illness and in their own bereavement
- uses a team approach to address the needs of patients and families, including bereavement counselling if indicated
- enhances the quality of life, and may also positively influence the course of illness
- is applicable early in the course of the illness, in conjunction with other therapies that are intended to prolong life, such as chemotherapy or radiotherapy, and includes those investigations needed to better understand and manage distressing clinical complications.[3]

Every person has the right to receive high-quality palliative care whatever the ill-health problems, regardless of the course and nature of the ill-health. The principles and philosophy of palliative care can be applied to any condition, irrespective of the clinical setting (see *Palliative Care within Mental health: principles and philosophy*). The goal of palliative care is to meet individual need and to provide the best quality of life for the person and their family. This approach includes physical, psychological, emotional, social and spiritual health, extending into bereavement, grief and loss, which can occur before, during and after death.

The philosophy and knowledge within the mental health and palliative care disciplines can be integrated, thus providing the very highest standard of care and practice for individuals experiencing health problems.

As in mental health, palliative care relies considerably on intra-/inter-disciplinary teamwork, an integral part of the philosophy of both disciplines, providing a responsive and sustained approach to person-centred care and practice.

RESPECTING LIFE

The mandate for palliative care offers a respect for life, and accepts the inevitability of death. Therefore treatment is balanced against its inherent burdens. Supportive medical measures used in acute situations, such as the use of intravenous infusions, the taking of blood gases, recording of blood pressure, artificial feeding, etc. is responsible practice (*see* Chapters 3 and 13). However, when there is an acknowledgement that there is going to be no return to good health, and/or the person is diagnosed as dying, this becomes inappropriate practice, and all measures possible to ensure freedom from distressing symptoms, physical and psychological, are maintained.[4]

Good communication is a prime function and fundamental within mental health and palliative care. The essence of good communication is our ability to listen carefully to what we are being told if the person is to feel fully heard and understood (*see* Chapter 15). It is not only about our interpretation of the information in order to manage complex needs and symptoms. It is about ensuring that we convey, with empathy, the validity of the person and their story.

Communication is imperative with and between the families, so that they are in no doubt about what we are doing (*see* Chapter 6). If we are to give the person free choices, then they must be properly informed about what those choices are, and the consequences of the choices they make. The individual is facing strong feelings and emotions as a direct consequence of her or his ill-health, such as anger, sadness, fear and anxiety, and is facing existential concerns, which demand exploration and sensitive approaches in order to reduce and allay the many and varied emotions experienced. Improved awareness of palliative care is a first step toward reducing disparities in utilisation of important and useful services for persons experiencing life-changing, life-limiting ill-health. Lack of awareness may limit access to needed palliative care.[5]

HUMANITY IN CARING

> Humanity is the place where you will find someone who will enter into
> your suffering and never leave you there alone.[6]

The human condition encompasses the experiences of being human. Human nature refers to certain characteristics that humans have in common: as human beings, we have certain characteristics, such as empathy, compassion, aggression and fear.

Being human is about the acceptance of every human being for just being another human being, regardless of colour, religion, race or gender (*see* Chapter 4 and *Palliative Care within Mental health: principles and philosophy* Chapters 3 and 9). When caring for people who are ill, we are constantly challenged to provide support and care in a human and compassionate way. The person-centred philosophy of mental health and palliative care is based on humanness and compassion. The focus is not just on the ill-health or the complex symptoms it produces, but is actively involved in finding out the needs of the whole person. In order to carry out this level of person-centred care, we must attend to the three indivisible facets of the human condition – the mind, body and spirit of humankind.[7]

THE ESSENCE OF CARING

Florence Nightingale[8] firmly believed that the essence of nursing rested on the nurse's capacity to provide humane, sensitive care to the sick, which she believed would allow healing. The therapeutic relationship in mental health has its origins in the work of Peplau,[9] who introduced her Theory of Interpersonal Relations, which focused on the human connection between the professional and individual. In today's healthcare environment, the human relationship is in danger of being overlooked in deference to computerised technology and financial restraints. We acknowledge the beneficial advantages of such technology – this registers the person's vital observations, but fails to provide information relevant to the person as a human being.[10]

> When John was very ill, I would sit with him for hours on end. The nurses
> would come into the room, check the computers, which noted his pulse,
> breathing and blood pressure, check his drip, and take blood when needed.
> They were very efficient in this respect, but they never really talked to him,
> asked him '*how*' he was feeling, or really talked to me. I was desperate for

someone to tell me what was happening – I thought he was dying – but no one said anything only that 'his obs [medical observations] are fine, he's just sleepy'. They concentrated on the technology, not on John as a person with feelings; they did not see his suffering. (Anon.)

WARMTH, COMPANIONSHIP AND ACCEPTANCE

Caring for someone should be a human activity – performed as humanly as possible, one person to another, on an equal footing. We meet people at a time of emotional need. However, do we have the resources to meet that need? Do we, in fact, see that there is an emotional need to be met? The difficult situations that we meet may tempt us to run away from the emotional pain – it is easier to deal with physical pain. In 'doing', rather than 'being' we can easily fail to reach the 'meaning' of the situation, a meaning which will offer an opportunity for us to discover how we can best help the person, in a compassionate way. We need to have a genuine desire to help, to acknowledge the pain of another, to make a human response.

SUFFERING

Suffering is subjective, encompassing factors which diminish quality of life, a perception of distress, and ultimately an expression of a life not worth living.[11] Suffering can be physical, emotional, spiritual, mental or all of these. Relief of suffering is an important goal for all professionals and a mutual commitment exists to reduce and relieve suffering. However, no type of care can ever alleviate *all* suffering, and some issues will always defy explanation. It is not only the person themselves who suffer, feeling isolated and desperate, but also the family and often the professional (*see* Chapters 5 and 15). Suffering is all-embracing; it affects us all. *It is part of life.*

A GENUINE DESIRE TO HELP

In order for us to try to help the person, we need to be fully present, to focus on the experience of that person – to listen fully to their story, for they will have one to tell, rather than be focused on ourselves, in order to protect us from the suffering of another. Watching someone suffer causes distress within ourselves and witnessing this suffering does not leave us untouched. As helpers we make human responses, showing compassion, empathy and understanding, and the offering of hope. We need the desire and competence to act, to acknowledge and share in the other's suffering and to make worthwhile and purposeful responses to the person's pain.

The family are important (*see* Chapter 5). Watching someone you love in physical and/or emotional pain and suffering causes distress that goes far beyond words.

I sat with Carrie for days, feeling very alone, although I was not alone. The family, her husband and child, were present and trying, as best as they could, to act as normally as possible, in a situation that was, to my mind, far from normal. Surgery had left her with complications. She was very ill, with fever and bad headaches as soon as she sat upright. Severe pain had been problematic for many months [*see* Chapter 8]. We had had to watch her then, a young woman, in the throes of motherhood, struggling to walk, to sleep, to play with her child. It had been impossible for her to do normal daily things. Things that we would all take for granted, basic easy tasks like cooking or washing up. Pain prevented any quality of life. There was also the emotional pain for her; I watched her dawning realisation that she had lost so much already; her assumed world had crumbled. All that she had looked forward to in the future had been taken away … what was there left? This, for me, was the most painful of all her suffering. The surgery seemed so futile, so I sat, alone in my desperation, not knowing how best to help, and feeling unheard by the visiting professionals. I wanted to shout; I was helpless to relieve any of her distress. I could not make it better for her. I felt I knew what should be done to help her suffering and to alleviate some of her physical and mental distress, but I sat alone, watching, waiting – until someone who recognised her physical and emotional pain, knew what needed to be done; listened to the family, managed the situation and changed the course of action. It only took one person to *see*, to *understand* and to *feel*. (Anon.)

The above is a brief extract of a mother's pain. Suffering affects the family as much as it does the sufferer, and as human beings we try to find a way to help support the whole family. We also have to be realistic! We may not be able to relieve the person's suffering, but we are trying our best, motivated in the purest way possible. Whatever we do, even if it is not ultimately successful, it cannot be thought of as detrimental, or harmful to that person.

SELF-KNOWING

As adults, we have the capacity to *feel* and to *think*, as well as the capacity to think about feelings. Being able to imagine the feelings of others is the cognitive basis for empathy.[12] It is helpful to be self-aware and 'knowing' oneself is the fundamental axiom in both mental health and palliative care. Self-awareness enriches our own understanding of *who* we are.

Possessing self-awareness indicates that we have a philosophical belief about life, death and the human condition.[13] It is important to examine our own beliefs in order to influence the way we interpret and make use of the person's story about him- or herself. When we have been touched, as human beings, by the pain of others, we may try to find strategies to distance ourselves from that pain, in order for us to survive, and move on to offer support to others within our care.

COMPASSION

Compassion becomes the dominant premise in the provision and conservation of care and practice and the art of caring lies in the relationship with the person, the family and is inclusive of our colleagues within the intra-/inter-disciplinary team (*see* Chapters 2 and 15). When offering a helping relationship, based on empathic understanding, it is important, as far as we can, to remain connected to that person. As we go through our own life, we learn to use our own experiences to help those we care for.[12] We all recognise and feel something about the benefits of compassion. In one way, we are all the same – we all want to avoid suffering. What, then, is *compassion* (see *Palliative Care within Mental health: principles and philosophy*, Chapter 6)? It is not simply a sense of sympathy or caring for the person suffering. Sogyal Rinpoche explains it as a sustained and practical determination to do whatever is possible and necessary to help alleviate the suffering of another.[14] Neither is it a sense of pity. Pity has its roots in fear, a sense of smugness, or arrogance. We need to move from pity to compassion. However, both sympathy and pity may be useful for a short period; both may bring some comfort to the sufferer during episodes of extreme suffering. At best, it is still an expression of sadness for the person who is suffering. It can also help to validate the person's suffering, as it can be so easy for a person's suffering to be minimised, for example, by being told to have a *positive attitude*!

> Nobody has much sympathy about my fear of taking so many tablets? This makes me feel undervalued and misunderstood. They say, it's this, or your life! I know that, and I don't need to be convinced. Of course I want my life, but they are just missing the point. (Anon.)

Compassion provides some indication of acceptance of the person's dilemma, it is strength-giving and affords comfort. This is not to say that feeling compassionate is easy. It is often challenging and difficult, and causes suffering for ourselves, as we share in the suffering of another.

> She [the nurse] sits quietly, nods as if she understands, holding my hand. It's so difficult and so complicated for you. We all feel for you and your children; it could be anyone of us … She stops; she gives full eye contact; it tells me, she knows; she understands. (Anon.)

Those we care for are our teachers. If we remain open, with a sense of allowingness, we can learn to develop our compassion for others. Each person we come into contact with who is ill, or who is dying, will teach us. *All we have to do is … listen and reflect.*

SUBSTANCE USE

The problems encountered by prolonged and excessive use of alcohol and other drugs (substance use) have an important consideration in the often long-term mental and physical health issues that accompany such use. Therefore we need to be open to the types of problems encountered and our role in offering palliative care to these individuals and family. Whilst Chapter 14 addresses some of these problems, the reader is asked to be open-minded throughout this book to the problems that arise because of substance use and/or existing mental health problems amongst the people we care for.

HOW TO

Before we can commence on any intervention and treatment programme we have to acknowledge that people are unique individuals, each with his or her own thoughts, feelings, needs, losses, loves … We need to own the philosophy that one size does *not* fit all. Whilst there may be some similarities in the approaches used and the symptom experienced, each person will need different interventions once these needs and expectations have been acknowledged. For example, pain for one person may be similar but the experience of pain is completely individual (*see* Chapter 8). Careful management and attention to detail is the key to improving the individual's experience and pain management. The person who complains of pain is not a weak person or a moaning person, but a unique individual with his or her own needs and expectations.

> Pain is what the patient says it is.[15]

To begin the process of care and practice we must first appreciate *how* we can maintain and influence compassion, respect and dignity for that individual (*see* Chapter 2). This may involve many problems along our path and maybe present us with numerous ethical dilemmas (Chapter 3), often a minefield for the individual, family and professional. People need supporting through the care but more importantly *after* the care; what happens next is our responsibility as the professional on whom people depend. Additionally, we need to be culturally competent to appreciate the individual needs of the person and family, so that we can incorporate those needs and expectations into our care and practice (*see* Chapter 4). This involves not just knowing but acting upon that knowledge at all times.

Each chapter recognises the needs and expectations of the family who are integral to the individuals needs and expectations (*see* Chapter 5). If we are to encompass the care and practice needs of the individual, we cannot do this without involving the family or friends acknowledged by the individual as significant to that person.

Dying at home is an emotive subject and a very subjective decision on the part of the person and the family (*see* Chapters 3, 6, 11 and 12). All must feel truly involved in the decision-making process and supported throughout the processes of prolonged ill-health and, just as importantly for the family, supported through and after the death of the individual. If the person wishes to die at home (*see* Chapter 6), and there is no essential reason why this cannot happen, then all steps must be taken to ensure the person's wish is met.

The professional cannot meet the needs of the individual or family without a thorough assessment (*see* Chapter 7). A quick five minutes is not enough! Having said that, assessment must be spread over time, as needs change, and not a one-off exercise to be 'done' before the professional moves on. Sitting with the person or family filling out forms does not constitute meaningful assessment. Such is perceived as impersonal and detached from that person's real life and needs.

The suicidal person needs compassionate care and open assessment and intervention in order to understand the needs of the individual. However, just as important are the needs of the family, who are often confused and distressed as to why the person feels the need to end his or her life and/or the progression and/or symptoms experienced by their loved ones (*see* Chapter 10, 13).

Long-term mental health problems bring a plethora of needs and expectations for the individual and family (Chapter 10). Life will need to be re-evaluated in order to incorporate the impact of the ill-health. Explanations as to what interventions are available, and seeing that someone 'cares' about them. Just as important is to ensure there is a network of support available to the person and family. If the person feels valued, then aiding him or her to accept something that has interfered with their life expectancy and future plans is integral to his or her daily living. A future can be achieved and a relatively stable path developed with safety nets in place when needed. However, these should not be merely reactive but proactive.

Dementia is traumatic to the individual and family (*see* Chapters 11 and 12). The loss of someone we love is experienced when the person is still alive, which brings the emotions of guilt and anger. The person in early stages of dementia may have some insight, which may be frightening, and they feel lost. Moreover, there may be embarrassment and a feeling of foolishness for the person experiencing dementia. To work alongside and encourage an active mind is essential as is 'cupping/holding' the family in their grief.

Euthanasia is emotive, and yet there is no medical path through this minefield. There are sound reasons why euthanasia should not be permitted and Chapter 13 addresses these in a meaningful and thought-provoking way.

CONCLUSION

Palliative care becomes important when we cannot offer a cure but can offer symptom management, but not total control. Therefore, it does apply to mental health and substance use problems. To some extent, mental health and substance use professionals may offer such an approach; however, we have a lot to learn from specialist palliative care professionals.

When we talked with mental health colleagues it was hard to get over that we were not talking about individuals experiencing mental health issues who also had a diagnosis of cancer – the concept was alien, and indeed ridiculed by some. The employer of one potential author would not permit her to write for the first book because 'it did not relate to mental health'. Clearly, a lot of work needs to be done before we can truly embrace the palliative care and practice philosophy. This is despite a growing awareness that a palliative care approach – in the true sense of the term – can be meaningful to the individual we have contact with on a daily basis. It offers hope, not of a cure, but that the professional is willing to work alongside the individual to manage symptoms that improve the quality of life for that individual and family.

Both books are a *beginning* and will need much building upon to influence changes in care, practice, behaviour and attitude of professionals. However, it can be done and costs nothing other than compassionate care and practice. Change can be achieved by working *with* the individual and family, taking time to understand and appreciate their collective problems, then acting to support, guide and improve each person's quality of life.

REFERENCES

1 Barker P, Buchanan-Barker P. Mental health in an age of celebrity: the courage to care. *Journal of Medical Ethics.* 2008; **34**: 110–4.
2 Saunders C. Care of the dying – the problem of euthanasia. *Nursing Times.* 1976; **1 July**: 1003–5.
3 World Health Organization. *WHO Definition of Palliative Care.* Geneva: WHO; 1990.
4 Twycross R. *Introducing Palliative Care.* 4th ed. Oxford: Radcliffe Publishing; 2002.
5 Matsuyama RK, Balliet W, Ingram K, *et al.* Will patients want hospice or palliative care if they do not know what it is? *Journal of Hospice and Palliative Nursing.* 2011; **13**: 41–6.
6 Roy DJ. Humanity: idea, image, reality. *Journal of Palliative Care.* 2004; **20**: 131–2.
7 Hopper A. Meeting the spiritual needs of patients through holistic practice. *European Journal of Palliative Care.* 2000; **7**: 60–3.
8 Nightingale F. *Notes of Nursing: what it is and what it is not.* Philadelphia: JP Lippincott; 1946.
9 Peplau, HE. The heart of nursing: interpersonal relations. *Canadian Nurse.* 1965; **61**: 273–5.
10 American Humanist Association. 2002. Available at: www.americanhumanist.org/humanism/ Humanism_Unmodified (accessed 14 November 2013).
11 Cherny NI, Coyle C, Foley KM. Suffering in the advanced cancer patient: a definition and taxonomy. *Journal of Palliative Care.* 1994; **10**: 57–70.
12 Lendrum S, Syme G. *Gift of Tears: a practical approach to loss and bereavement in counselling and psychotherapy.* 2nd ed. East Sussex: Routledge; 2004.
13 Eckroth-Bucher M. Philosophical basis and practice of self-awareness in psychiatric nursing. *Journal of Psychosocial Nursing.* 2001; **39**: 32–9.
14 Rinpoche S. *The Tibetan Book of Living and Dying: a spiritual classic from one of the foremost interpreters of Tibetan Buddhism to the West.* Classic ed. London: Rider; 2008.
15 McCaffery M. *Nursing Practice Theories related to Cognition, Bodily Pain, and Man–Environment Interactions.* Los Angeles: University of California at Los Angeles Student Store; 1968. p. 95.

TO LEARN MORE

- Cooper DB, Cooper J, editors. *Palliative Care within Mental Health: principles and philosophy.* London/New York: Radcliffe Publishing; 2012.

CHAPTER 2

Compassion, respect and dignity

David B Cooper

DEFINITIONS

➤ **Compassion:** a feeling of deep sympathy and sorrow for another who is stricken by misfortune, accompanied by a strong desire to alleviate the suffering.[1]

➤ **Respect:** esteem for, or a sense of, the worth or excellence of a person, a personal quality or ability, or something considered as a manifestation of a personal quality or ability.[2]

➤ **Dignity:** bearing, conduct or speech indicative of self-respect or appreciation of the formality or gravity of an occasion or situation.[3]

REFLECTIVE PRACTICE EXERCISE 2.1

Time: 10 minutes

The words 'compassion', 'respect' and 'dignity' are often used in health and social care, but in an abstract sense as they are difficult to define. There is an understanding amongst us that we know what they mean and that we provide compassion, respect and dignity in the care that we give.

● Think carefully about the last shift you worked.
● Note 'how' you acted with compassion, respect and dignity.
● What did you achieve?

INTRODUCTION

Compassion, respect and dignity are subjective; they are about being with the person and family, as well as professional colleagues and friends – one human being to another – seeing through the other person's eyes and empathising with that person's pain, fear, joy, loss or sadness. We cannot truly be that person, but we can offer ourselves in the way we would expect to receive from others – treating people as you would wish for yourself and your family. Regardless of our work role and/or environment, we should be treating the person and family as if they were invited guests into our home.

Compassion is not about pity – although pity may be helpful to the person and family in the short term as it may add some comfort in a time of need – it is a stage beyond that, to where we embrace the person with warmth and understanding, being non-judgemental. I think I know what dignity is and hope that I treat others with dignity and respect. However, reflecting on this it is very difficult to translate these feeling into words.

To be clear about the person's and family's understanding of what dignity is, we need to ask them what their perception of dignity is – what it means to them – from this, we can explore the extent of their loss of dignity.[4]

An enquiry into the Mid-Staffordshire NHS Foundation Trust (UK) reported a general lack of care and compassion towards the individuals in need of that care.[5] Examples of lack of compassion, dignity and respect included:

➤ dependent individuals being left in bed to urinate and/or defecate because either there was no one available to take the person to the bathroom or no one responded after the request for a commode was made
➤ incidents of callous uncaring treatment towards the individual
➤ dependent people being left unwashed in bed
➤ dependent people being left without food or fluids if they needed help
➤ prescribed medication being omitted.[5]

SELF-ASSESSMENT EXERCISE 2.1

Time: 5 minutes
Make a list of what you value most from others – your views of compassion, respect and dignity.

A review of the year 2012/2013 by one National Health Service (NHS – UK) Trust formally listed their view on dignity, compassion and respect as:[6]

➤ valuing the person as an individual
➤ working with a can-do attitude, no matter how large or small the request or task, in everything we do
➤ responding with humanity and kindness. This involves purposefully looking for what we can do or what can be done without waiting to be asked
➤ taking full responsibility and accountability for our actions, omissions, decisions and behaviour.[6]

SELF-ASSESSMENT EXERCISE 2.2

Time: 15 minutes
- What would it take for you to maintain a change in attitude and behaviour in your workplace?
- How could you become a change agent, ensuring that caring and compassionate attitudes become as important as knowledge and skills?

It would be an excellent world if we as professionals always treated people with compassion, respect and dignity. Sadly we do not – we all have failings when caring for individuals and their family. Yet compassion, respect and dignity cost nothing and have no financial impact on the service. The cost is to ourselves – just a moment in time to understand a person's pain and/or to empathise with the family who have lost a loved one. We acknowledge that there is a huge amount of paperwork to get through and the computer records need updating, but these are things that need to be done in the matter of course. Showing compassion, respect and dignity – humanity – can work alongside these tasks. They involve merely being human and demonstrating humanness toward others.

KEY POINT 2.1

We all need to pay attention to our attitudes of caring.

The case studies below are real; the professionals' action affected the individuals and the families. All these individuals were dying and in hospital. David had a diagnosis of carcinoma of the lung with secondaries in the bone and was in the last three days of his life. Charlie had a cardiovascular accident (CVA – stroke); he was mostly unconscious and had little awareness when semi-conscious. Joyce had B-cell lymphoma with lung and bone secondaries. For Charlie and Joyce – we *were* the family.

Case Study 2.1 – David

David (59) was in the terminal stages of cancer. He was alert and was experiencing severe pain. His treatment was active and the family and David had not been made aware of his diagnosis. The family did, however, suspect that David was indeed dying and requested a palliative care assessment from the hospital-based Macmillan nurse for recommendations as to how David should be treated at this stage in his ill-health. The only way to make a referral was through David's consultant. However, the consultant felt David 'did not need specialist palliative care'.

Three days before David's death he was in obvious uncontrolled pain ... the nurse had left a medicine pot containing Oramorph on David's bedside table, however, he had not been advised as to what it was or indeed that he should take it. The family spoke with the nurse about David's pain and asked for pain relief for him. It was at this stage the nurse relayed the information that his analgesia was the liquid in the pot on his table! As David went to pick up the medicine pot he accidentally tipped it over ... most of the contents absorbed into a tissue on David's table. This was explained to the nurse who checked the medication sheet and advised the family David could not have any further pain relief as he 'was not due' any medication for another 2 hours. The nurse ignored the family's plea that he had not been able to take the current medication because of spillage ... but the drug chart had been signed for that dose and consequently David could not have any more!

Twenty-four hours before his death it was acknowledged that David needed to be treated palliatively ... but that decision was too late! The specialist palliative care nurse would have been able to assess David's pain, offering expertise as to the amount of analgesia needed to manage David's severe pain.

In the above case study, David's requests for pain relief were completely ignored, as were those of the family. The inaction on the consultant's part was that he knew about the 'patient' so why did David need referral to a specialist palliative care nurse? The nurse's inaction regarding the analgesia spillage and lack of adequate pain control related merely to a piece of paper and the signature, not the actual situation and David's need for severe pain management.

SELF-ASSESSMENT EXERCISE 2.3

Time: 10 minutes
- How would you have managed this situation?
- For the family?
- For David?

Case Study 2.2 – Charlie – Part I

Charlie was in the intensive care unit a few hours after his CVA. The paraphernalia and tubes, drips and so on were disturbing to the family and no explanation was given as to the equipment or indeed what could be expected of them when the nurse was absent.

The family were called into a room where the consultant suggested that little more could be done for Charlie and he needed to be treated palliatively. Consequently, Charlie was to be moved to a sister site to be cared for. When the family arrived, it became clear that the ward was an acute medical ward and the family were told that the consultant 'did not believe in palliative care'. So intensive treatment continued, despite the family's request for a specialist palliative care assessment.

Here was a complete lack of communication from one consultant to another. The family's agreement with palliative care was completely ignored and they were left feeling helpless and vulnerable through the dying process of some four weeks. The consultant was a mystical figure whose messages were given by others; the family did not see the consultant at all!

Case Study 2.2 – Charlie – Part II

Charlie was being treated actively and was on an intravenous drip. He was unconscious and non-responsive. The family were seated two at each side of Charlie, holding his hands. The nurse entered the room and immediately went to the drip/drip stand, checked the levels and speed, and then left the room. At no time did she acknowledge Charlie or his family … it was as if they were non-existent … the important thing was the drip!

SELF-ASSESSMENT EXERCISE 2.4

Time: 5 minutes

What would you have done differently to make this encounter therapeutically beneficial for Charlie and his family?

KEY POINT 2.2

The elements of compassion, respect and dignity were missing.

Case Study 2.2 – Charlie – Part III

A couple of days after transfer to the acute ward Charlie was restless, unable to communicate his distress, or to say if he was in pain. The family advised the nurses that Charlie had a known prostate problem and had difficulty passing urine. This guidance from the family was not acted upon until Charlie was dying. Eventually, a catheter was inserted.

Whilst semi-conscious but non-responsive Charlie was given an effective laxative. The following day, though unconscious, Charlie was passing loose stools. This was drawn to the attention of the nurses, who after a while came and changed Charlie's bed. This happened again and the family advised the nurses accordingly, the nurses were visibly unhappy with this information and left Charlie in his own faeces, despite reminders from his family, for several hours. On neither of the above occasions did the nurses acknowledge the family in the room or address Charlie to advise him of what was happening.

Case Study 2.2 – Charlie – Part IV

Approximately one week before Charlie's death the family again visited him. On entering the ward Charlie was unconscious. He had a large haematoma on his head which had been sutured, an open cut to his nose and evidence of a nose bleed. Later exploration noted bruising on Charlie's arms and knees.

A family member went to ask what had happened. The ward sister accompanied the relative to the bedside, did not draw the curtains, and stated: 'I had hoped to catch you before you came in'! The family were advised that Charlie had been lifted out of his bed and sat on a bedside commode ... he had subsequently been left there whilst the nurse went to attend another person. On hearing a loud 'thud', the nurse returned to find Charlie on the floor.

When challenged by the family as to who would place an unconscious person on a bedside commode, they were advised it was usual practice 'as we do not want him to mess his bed ... do we? It could lead to bedsores!'

The family were unable to ascertain who the nurse was that had undertaken this task, but during the day staff nurses and healthcare assistants came over and expressed their regret and stated openly that it should not have happened. The family therefore deduced that the person who had placed Charlie on the commode was the ward sister, though when challenged this was denied. Despite a formal complaint, nothing was done! Several days later, Charlie died.

Case Study 2.2 happened to one person and his family, and demonstrates common breaches of compassion, respect and dignity. It would be helpful to say these were the only examples of the poor care Charlie and his family received. Sadly, they were not. Indeed, it appeared to be common practice on this ward. When a whole system fails, it is time to examine who and what is to blame and introduce re-education strategies. It has been observed that nurses below the ward manager/sister generally take a lead on the quality of care given – or not given – from the person in charge.

KEY POINT 2.3

Good quality and standard of care stems from the ward sister downward, who leads by example.

Case Study 2.2 – Charlie – Part V

Charlie did not die peacefully. His death was made worse for him and his family by the lack of compassion, respect and dignity that they all experienced. It was only the day before Charlie died that it was acknowledged that Charlie was indeed dying and the family's request for the palliative care nurse was taken on board. The nurse attended the ward the next day ... but it was too late for Charlie.

Prior to his death Charlie had been experiencing terminal restlessness – a situation that can be managed by appropriate medication and explanations. His death was distressing not only for Charlie but also his family, who had to stand by helplessly and observe Charlie's distress. It was not a good death.

Case Study 2.3 – Joyce

Joyce (74) was diagnosed with terminal cancer and had fluid on her lungs and failure to retain oxygen at normal levels. The consultant had insisted in front of Joyce and the family that Joyce merely had a severe chest infection! It was only two days before her death that Joyce was properly diagnosed with B-cell lymphoma with bone and lung secondaries, and it was acknowledged that Joyce was dying.

The senior house officer made the decision that Joyce should wear a full-face pressurised oxygen mask. He was unaware that Joyce had always been claustrophobic. On the family's arrival Joyce looked fearful. When asked what the matter was she stated she did not want the mask – it was frightening her and she felt she could not breathe. It transpired that neither Joyce nor her family had given consent and the senior house officer assumed that it was okay. Because the doctor 'said so' Joyce was afraid to question this in case of reprisals from the staff for her being 'awkward'. When confronted by a relative the doctor acknowledged that indeed he had not asked Joyce for her permission. The relative, a nurse, insisted that the doctor go and ask Joyce what '*she*' wanted. When the doctor asked Joyce, she stated that she 'did not like it' and 'I do not want it on'. The mask was removed.

Two days before her death Joyce received specialist palliation for her intractable symptoms and died peacefully in her sleep.

Common breaches of compassion, respect and dignity are:

➤ leaving the curtain screen open with a half-dressed person in bed
➤ leaving the person on the commode for too long and with no way of calling for help
➤ relaying bad news behind the curtain with only the curtain for privacy
➤ ignoring relatives and the person when undertaking a procedure
➤ failing to answer direct questions from the person and family
➤ hiding behind 'official' procedures
➤ hiding behind a uniform.

This list is by no means exhaustive but is a view of just a few basic things that we can all change.

CONCLUSION

Speaking from experience, no one is perfect! We have all been involved in situations that should not have been. We need to learn from our failings – and not just from the good – so that our practice in the care of the individual, the family and each other develops and becomes meaningful to those who are within our care. The ability to give compassionate, respectful care with dignity is within all of us, we merely need to look for it and put this into practice when caring for the person and his or her family.

As discussed above, this is not about the lack of time or the number of professionals on duty. Whilst these can impact on our ability to offer care, they cannot, and should not, affect our ability to offer compassion, respect and dignity.

For compassion, respect and dignity to be a 'normal' attitude, it requires a change in our attitudes and the desire to maintain this fundamental attitudinal change and attention to the smallest detail. For this to happen, the demonstration of compassion, respect and dignity must come from the top down in health and social care. This is the only way compassion, respect and dignity can be passed on to junior members of the intra-/inter-disciplinary team.

REFERENCES

1 Dictionary.com. Available at: http://dictionary.reference.com/browse/compassion (accessed 26 February 2014).
2 Dictionary.com. Available at: http://dictionary.reference.com/browse/respect (accessed 26 February 2014).
3 Dictionary.com. Available at: http://dictionary.reference.com/browse/dignity (accessed 26 February 2014).
4 Jeffrey J. *Patient-centred Ethics and Communication at the End of Life*. Oxford/Seattle: Radcliffe Publishing; 2006. p. 25.
5 Tinge J. Francis Report highlights issues of patients safety in hospital. *British Journal of Nursing*. 2013; **22**: 238–9.
6 Surrey and Sussex Healthcare NHS Trust. *Review of Last Year (2012/2013) and our Priorities for This Year (2013/2014)*. Redhill: Surrey and Sussex Healthcare NHS Trust; 2013. p. 7.

CHAPTER 3

Overcoming ethical dilemmas

Cynthia MA Geppert

The world is full of suffering; it is also full of overcoming it.[1]

MENTAL HEALTH AND PALLIATIVE CARE ETHICS: TWO WORLDS

This groundbreaking volume represents a pioneering effort to synchronise the orbits of two worlds of theory and practice that have often proceeded on isolated, even at times antagonistic, trajectories: mental health and palliative care. As a mental health ethicist consulting in a large hospital with an aging population with multiple medical and mental health comorbidities, I have personally encountered the clash of these two worlds ... and how poorly their discord serves individuals, families and professionals. Bioethics is for me, and I believe for many of you, our fellow professionals from both worlds, a means of closing the divide between our respective universes. In this chapter, I endeavour to present some case-based best practice strategies from palliative care and humanistic ethics that can enable mental health and palliative care professionals to travel beyond their own traditions and training. However, first we must understand some of the conceptual gaps in ethical assumptions that separate us, outlined in Table 3.1.

TABLE 3.1 Comparison of mental health and palliative care ethical assumptions

Assumption	Mental health	Palliative care
Orientation	• Biobehavioural	• Humanistic
Objectives	• Cure disease • Control symptoms	• Improve quality of life • Relieve suffering
Focus	• Individual person	• Person, family, community
Autonomy	• Constraint and compulsion if needed to prevent harm	• Choice and flexibility even if reduces length of life

ARTIFICIAL NUTRITION AND HYDRATION IN DEMENTIA: A PARADIGM CASE FOR MENTAL HEALTH PALLIATIVE ETHICS

SELF-ASSESSMENT EXERCISE 3.1

Time: 45 minutes

Decisions regarding the use of artificial nutrition and hydration in persons experiencing advanced dementia are perhaps the most agonising ethical dilemmas families and professionals living and working at the intersection of mental health and palliative care confront.[2]

Read the case scenario below carefully:

- consider your current clinical knowledge and skill in responding to the clinical and psychosocial aspects of the case
- articulate and reflect on the values and emotions the case raises for you as a professional and a human being
- after you have read the chapter, revisit this exercise and see if your understanding or attitudes have changed.

Case Study 3.1 – Mary, faith and food

Mary is an 82-year-old widow with advanced Alzheimer dementia. Mary had been doing fairly well in a nursing home specialising in dementia care for four years. Over the last six months, she has lost interest in eating, even when family brings in favourite foods. She has now lost 25 pounds and seems to have some difficulty swallowing, which has led to repeated bouts of pneumonia. These have always responded well to antibiotics and Mary has recovered, although never quite back to where she was before the acute ill-health. The professionals at the care home believe it is in Mary's best medical interest to be transferred to hospital for an evaluation of her anorexia and weight loss and consideration of artificial nutrition and hydration. Multiple specialists examine Mary and diagnose her with dysphagia and adult failure to thrive. They recommend placement of a percutaneous gastric tube (PEG) to supply adequate nutrition and to reduce aspiration risk. Mary had executed an advance directive 10 years ago when first diagnosed with dementia and indicated her preference for life-sustaining medical treatment so long as she had a good quality of life. Mary's two sons believe their mother has reached the point where she can barely interact and has little to enjoy and the PEG tube will only prolong her discomfort. Mary's youngest daughter, Eileen, is named as the official healthcare proxy and has been her main caregiver. Like her mother, she is a devout Catholic who believes it is a sin to allow her mother to starve to death.

Chapter themes

This case scenario is one of the most distressing and controversial dilemmas in palliative care and mental health, and introduces many of the core themes of the chapter and the book, such as the family as the unit of care, spirituality and quality of life issues. Resolution of the ethical dilemma here will not be possible without the collaboration of a intra-/inter-disciplinary team of professionals working in tandem with Mary's family and her other important relationships toward a shared goal of providing respectful and compassionate person-centred care (*see* Chapters 11, 12).

INTRODUCTION

This chapter is not just about ethical dilemmas, but is more significantly about overcoming them. However, before we can overcome a dilemma, we must be able to recognise one and differentiate it from other types of salient concerns such as clinical, legal, cultural and social. A good working definition of an ethical dilemma useful for general practice comes from Professor Braunack-Mayer:

> Ethical dilemmas, however, are defined rather more narrowly, as situations in which, on moral grounds, persons ought both to do and not to do something. Such a definition implies that issues of conflict and choice are central to moral dilemmas.[3]

A true ethical dilemma, then, involves a conflict between two or more important ethical values or principles. An ethical dilemma usually involves a choice between two ethical courses of action, one of which may prevent the other from being realised. Ethical awareness is the ability to identify dilemmas and use ethical models and methods to resolve the dilemma through a process of prioritising, balancing, reconciling and specifying the salient values, principles and duties. As it does with clinical medicine, the use of a deliberate and reflective process can help professionals formulate an ethical differential diagnosis and prescription. A number of serviceable approaches[4,5,6] have been developed to provide a structure for professionals in analysing ethical dilemmas. Employing these models, especially in the challenging situations that arise in palliative mental health care, can help organise information to:

➤ prevent missing key pieces of the puzzle
➤ illuminate bias and ignorance that could prejudice judgements
➤ ensure all stakeholders and perspectives are included fairly
➤ place valid emotional, spiritual, cultural and social claims in a reasoned framework.

The most widely utilised and practical healthcare decision-making matrix is the four-box method of Jonsen, Winslade and Siegler outlined in Table 3.2.[7]

TABLE 3.2 Four-box method

Medical indications	*Person preferences*
• Diagnosis and prognosis	• Known wishes and values of the person
• Treatment plan	• Decisional capacity of person
• Medical goals	• Advance directive
	• Surrogates and standards of judgement
Quality of life	*Contextual features*
• Prospects for recovery	• Relationship connectedness
• Personal meaning in life	• Family conflicts
• Deficits from therapy	• Cultural and religious beliefs and practices
• Professional bias about quality of life	• Legal considerations
	• Conflicts of interest

REFLECTIVE PRACTICE EXERCISE 3.1 FOUR-BOX METHOD

> **Time: 20 minutes**
> • Draw and label the four boxes as shown in Table 3.2.
> • Work through Case Study 3.1 above by placing the issues and problems presented in the case in the appropriate boxes.
> • Compare your analysis to the example Table 3.4 at the end of this chapter (*see* p. 29).

Analysis of the basic areas of ethical concern is the platform on which a discussion with all involved parties and their respective preferences and interests can be combined to overcome the dilemmas in the case. However, what does overcoming mean in a bioethics case? The dictionary definition of 'overcoming' that fits best is 'to prevail over or surmount' difficulties. Each member of the family and professional team has a crucial part to play in this effort, and if all viewpoints are not solicited and respected then it is more likely that the result will fit with two other definitions of overcoming:
1 'to defeat another in conflict or competition' or
2 'to overpower as with emotion'.[8]

Even the finest advance care planning cannot predict all circumstances or prevent all conflict. Crucial to overcoming ethical dilemmas in the positive sense is utilising a palliative care or ethics consultation service, or both, to facilitate the discussion. Key points (3.1) of a constructive discussion of Mary's case and some of the core skills needed to make them are summarised below.

KEY POINT 3.1

Palliative-ethics discussion (*see* Case Study 3.1 to refresh your thinking p. 20)
• **Communication** – the professionals should explain to Eileen and her family that the percutaneous endoscopic gastrostomy (PEG) tube will not prevent Mary from aspirating.

- **Consistency** – all the professionals involved need to be on the same page in informing the family that the research on PEG tubes in dementia shows that in general the burdens outweigh the benefits.[9]
- **Coherence** – the professionals should diligently inquire into Mary's life and values history[10] to understand the context of the preferences expressed in the advance directive. This will likely require widening the circle of informants to friends and especially Mary's primary caregivers in the nursing home.
- **Clarification** – Eileen is expressing her religious belief that Catholicism requires her to ensure her mother receives artificial nutrition and hydration. No progress can be made without a chaplain or other clergy who can provide pastoral counselling on the Church's true position on this issue.[11]
- **Cultural competence** – the professionals should be sensitive to the symbolic and communal meaning of food and water as life sustenance and the stigma associated with starvation and deprivation (*see* Chapter 4).
- **Compassion** – the professionals should empathise with the moral distress of Eileen, her brothers and the other professionals caring for Mary and provide ongoing support (*see* Chapter 2).
- **Caring** – Mary and her brothers as well as staff at the care home may feel much more comfortable knowing they can hand-feed Mary bites of her favourite foods.

SELF-ASSESSMENT EXERCISE 3.2

Time: 30 minutes
- Review the difficult ethical dilemmas encountered in palliative mental health care in Table 3.3.
- Reflect on your own practice, and how many of these dilemmas you have faced.
- Of those you have not yet confronted, which do you think would be most problematic for you as a professional?
- Ask yourself why these particular situations are challenging. How can you enhance your ability to deal with them in the future?

TABLE 3.3 Difficult ethical dilemmas in palliative mental health

---

- Sex between residents with dementia in nursing homes.[12]
- The duty to warn as it applies to genetic testing for Huntington's disease and other dementias.[13]
- Appropriateness of palliative care as an option in anorexia nervosa.[14]
- Do Not Resuscitate (DNR) orders in persons who attempt suicide.[15]
- Application of futility criteria to advanced stages of mental ill-health.[16]
- Use of terminal sedation for existential distress.[17]

See references cited in this table to learn more about these issues.

Case Study 3.2 – Human immunodeficiency virus (HIV), confidentiality, capacity and consent

Raj (46) is experiencing bipolar I disorder and HIV. He immigrated to the UK from India 15 years earlier. His periods of mania and depression, as well as difficulty holding down a job, have adversely affected Raj's ability to adhere to the demanding regimen of highly active antiretroviral therapy and associated prophylactic medications he must take to control the virus. Raj collapses at a local market and is rushed to hospital, where he is diagnosed with acquired immunodeficiency syndrome (AIDS) and reactivated tuberculosis (TB).

Raj has been with his partner Duncan for the last seven years, but they never completed an advance directive. However, as Raj became sicker they had many conversations in which Raj made clear he did not want to be resuscitated if his heart or breathing stopped. Raj's parents are in India and he has sporadic contact with his brother, Sanjeev, who is an engineer studying in England. Raj never disclosed to his brother either his sexual orientation or that he was HIV positive for fear he would reject him and tell his parents. Raj was coherent enough when he was admitted to tell the physician that he wanted Duncan to be his surrogate. When Raj is admitted, the social worker contacts his brother, rather than his partner of seven years.

Soon after admission, Raj developed delirium and did not regain sufficient capacity to express his wishes. Duncan wants to take Raj home to die with hospice support. However, Sanjeev insists that Raj receive aggressive treatment, including forced mental health medications and life support if necessary to treat the TB, HIV and bipolar disorder. The professionals empathise with both Raj and Duncan, yet they know that without an advance directive and with no other family involved, Sanjeev could be the rightful surrogate. When they do try to remind Sanjeev of what Raj said when admitted, he responds that between the bipolar disorder and HIV, Raj could not have had the capacity to make any decisions.

REFLECTIVE PRACTICE EXERCISE 3.2

Time: 30 minutes
- Carefully review Case Study 3.2 in light of what you have learned so far in the chapter/book.
- Write down or type what you think the key points (3.2) are for this case, in terms of the following broad concepts:
  - confidentiality
  - capacity
  - consent.
- On your own, analyse the case using the four-box method for extra practice (*see* Table 3.2, p. 22).

KEY POINT 3.2

- **Confidentiality** – The social worker likely acted in good faith, and according to protocol, when she notified the next-of-kin. However, in a society that is increasingly diverse, professionals need to be aware of the many permutations of what related-ness and family can mean for an individual.

- **Confidentiality** – Even in liberal democracies like the US, UK and Australia, there is still considerable social stigma attached to mental health problems, to death and dying, and to homosexuality, especially in more traditional groups. Professionals need to be attuned to their own biases and those of the setting in which they practice and develop preventive ethics strategies to protect the rights and dignity of those marginalised. Raj likely would not have wished his lifestyle and ill-health to be disclosed to his brother.

- **Confidentiality** – Precisely because of the stigma attached to mental health problems and dependence disorders and to HIV, in many jurisdictions there is a higher level of privacy protection for these types of health information. Professionals need to know the rules and regulations applicable in their practice setting.

- **Capacity** – Even among professionals there is a prevailing myth that individuals with serious mental health problems like bipolar disorder or dementia are unable to make their own decisions.[18] While these disorders certainly can diminish the ability to reason regarding complicated medical situations or appreciate the full import of a decision, most individuals experiencing psychotic disorders and mild to moderate dementia can make their own decisions when professionals are patient, kind and innovative in framing the information.

- **Capacity** – Decision-making capacity is neither all-or-nothing, nor is it monolithic.[18] The ability to identify an individual that a person trusts and loves is elemental, and even an individual who is critically ill, like Raj, or one who has marked cognitive impairment can choose the person they would like to make decisions on their behalf.

- **Capacity** – This is a medical judgement, so it is the opinion of the professionals caring for Raj, not his brother, that determines whether or not he is able to communicate a preference for a surrogate.

- **Consent** – Informed consent is both a legal and ethical doctrine, but without an advance directive that expressly documents Raj's wishes, in many jurisdictions, legally Sanjeev is the decision-maker. It is hard to not argue ethically that the professionals should proceed on what Raj told the admitting physician he wanted.[19]

- **Consent** – While legally Sanjeev may be the surrogate, and this may intimidate professionals into following his instructions, even the surrogate is obligated to exercise substituted judgement, that is to 'make decisions as the individual would want them made if capable'. Duncan is the person in the best position to tell the surrogate and professionals about Raj's values and preferences and these must be respected and followed to the extent possible.[20]

PALLIATIVE MENTAL HEALTH CARE

Providing palliative mental health care will require realignment of the fundamental ethical assumptions that opened this chapter. The recovery movement[21] shares many of the principles of palliative care philosophy and offers a possible avenue of rapprochement between the two disciplines. Some bold thinkers are adopting palliative care models of care for treatment-resistant advanced stages of mental health problems.[22] The authors of this innovative proposal recognise that many individuals, families and professionals trained in a model of treatment in which severity of ill-health is directly correlated with aggressiveness of intervention may find the palliative approach morally distressing, equating it with giving up on the person and giving in to the disorder.

> Palliative approaches definitely should not be equated with the abandonment of hope or care but with a reformulation of goals. Setting meaningful and attainable goals may increase hope and reinforce effort, whereas actively chasing a sequence of failed treatments can lead to hopelessness via recurrent failure.[22]

The ethical axioms underpinning the model are abridged below.

Ethical axioms of the new philosophy[22]

➤ Reconfiguration of purpose of treatment away from cure toward care.
➤ Tailoring treatment to the needs and wishes of individuals and families.
➤ Individualising the treatment plan so it is responsive to changes in context and condition.
➤ Greater emphasis on social support and family psycho-education than on active neuropsychiatric treatment.
➤ Reducing burdensome side effects.
➤ Weighing risk–benefit profile of treatments with non-maleficence as the prime directive.
➤ Controlling symptoms that are either distressing or interfere with functioning.
➤ Goal is not remission of the disorder but recovery of quality of life.

SELF-ASSESSMENT EXERCISE 3.3

Time: 15 minutes
How such a meeting of the minds might reshape the ethics of caring for persons in the latter stage of mental ill-health is depicted in the third vignette (*see* Case Study 3.3).
● Before reading the final case, imagine three ways in which palliative care principles and practice could be adapted for the betterment of mental health treatment.
● Then think about your own work and list three aspects of your clinical practice where a palliative care approach could be adopted.
● See whether any of your ideas for improvement are reflected in the case.

Case Study 3.3 – The future of palliative mental health care

Robert (65) is experiencing chronic schizophrenia. He has lived his entire adult life with his parents, who are now in their eighties and in declining health. He has never been able to hold down a job or have a significant relationship. He has been in and out of mental institutions, both voluntarily and under commitment, although he has never been violent. Robert has tried numerous psychotropic medications, electroconvulsive therapy (ECT) and a variety of psychosocial interventions but none has effectuated a substantive improvement in his disorder.

As he has grown older, the positive symptoms of paranoia and hallucinations have become less commanding, but the negative symptoms have interfered more with his ability to function. Robert spends his weekdays in a programme for persons with serious mental ill-health and tries to help his parents with the house and yard on weekends. His dependence on nicotine has resulted in chronic obstructive pulmonary disease but Robert does not like to wear oxygen because it interferes with smoking, which is his biggest pleasure. Decades of antipsychotics have given Robert diabetes and obesity that he struggles to control with medication. Robert has been asking his parents for months if he can stop taking all the medications. Robert's psychiatrist, medical doctor and case manager are absolutely against his request and advise Robert and his parents that this would be tantamount to abandoning hope and even hint that this could be considered abuse of a vulnerable individual. The case manager points out that technically Robert is decisionally capable. The psychiatrist thinks that Robert is not depressed but misguided, and urges Robert and his parents to let him arrange admission to a clinical trials unit of the University Hospital in a large city 300 miles away. His parents long ago gave up their dreams for Robert to live a normal life.

After a lot of thought, Robert's parents agree with his request and inform the mental health care staff at the community clinic, 'we will not be around much longer and we worry what will happen to Robert when we are gone. If there is any chance he could be happy, even for a little while, after all he has lost, we have to take it'. Robert's sister is a nurse and is able to arrange for enrolment in a psychiatric palliative care residential programme that uses alternative treatments to treat refractory advanced mental ill-health.

Robert enjoys the pet and music therapy provided at the facility and seems calmer and more engaged when he returns home. Robert is even able to reduce his smoking using acupuncture and loses some weight working in the programme garden. The hallucinations do return off the antipsychotics, but so does more energy and insight that enable Robert to manage the voices through meditation.

CONCLUSION

This chapter began with a lamentation of the distance between the mental health and palliative care communities and practices, and ends with rejoicing over the advent of avenues of confluence through bioethics. The chapter has provided those professionals endeavouring to bridge the gap with a method of ethical decision making to navigate the dilemmas encountered along the way. A log of some of the common ethical dilemmas that cannot be overcome without closure of the divide between mental health and palliative care, and a set of questions, issues and resources to serve as a check and guide for the reorientation.

REFERENCES

1　Helen Keller. *Optimism*. New York: TY Crowell & Co.; 1903.
2　Geppert CM, Andrews MR, Druyan ME. Ethical issues in artificial nutrition and hydration: a review. *Journal of Parenteral and Enteral Nutrition*. 2010; **34**: 79–88.
3　Braunack-Mayer AJ. What makes a problem an ethical problem? An empirical perspective on the nature of ethical problems in general practice. *Journal of Medical Ethics*. 2001; **27**: 98–103. p. 98.
4　Kuhl DR, Wilensky P. Decision making at the end of life: a model using an ethical grid and principles of group process. *Journal of Palliative Medicine*. 1999; **2**: 75–86.
5　Hundert EM. A model for ethical problem solving in medicine, with practical applications. *American Journal of Psychiatry*. 1987; **144**: 839–46.
6　Markkula Center for Applied Ethics. *A Framework for Ethical Thinking*. Santa Clara, CA: Santa Clara University; 2009 [updated May 2009; cited 16 October 2010]. Available from: www.scu.edu/ethics/practicing/decision/framework.html (accessed 12 November 2013).
7　Jonsen AR, Seigler M, Winslade WJ. *Clinical Ethics: A Practical Approach to Ethical Decisions in Clinical Medicine*. 7th ed. New York: McGraw-Hill; 2010.
8　*The American Heritage Dictionary of the English Language*. 4th ed. Boston, MA: Houghton Mifflin; 2006.
9　Cervo FA, Bryan L, Farber S. To PEG or not to PEG: a review of evidence for placing feeding tubes in advanced dementia and the decision-making process. *Geriatrics*. 2006; **61**: 30–5.
10　Gibson JM, Lambert P, Nathanson P. The values history: an innovation in surrogate medical decision-making. *Law Medicine Health Care*. 1990; **18**: 202–12.
11　Sulmasy DP. Are feeding tubes morally obligatory? *St Anthony Messenger*. 2006; **January**: 28–32.
12　Mahieu L, Gastmans C. Sexuality in institutionalized elderly persons: a systematic review of argument-based ethics literature. *International Psychogeriatrics*. 2012; **24**: 346–57.
13　Hakimian R. Disclosure of Huntington's disease to family members: the dilemma of known but unknowing parties. *Genetic Testing*. 2000; **4**: 359–64.
14　Lopez A, Yager J, Feinstein RE. Medical futility and psychiatry: palliative care and hospice care as a last resort in the treatment of refractory anorexia nervosa. *International Journal of Eating Disorders*. 2010; **43**: 372–7.
15　Cook R, Pan P, Silverman R, *et al.* Do-not-resuscitate orders in suicidal patients: clinical, ethical, and legal dilemmas. *Psychosomatics*. 2010; **51**: 277–82.
16　Cholbi MJ. The terminal, the futile, and the psychiatrically disordered. *International Journal of Law and Psychiatry*. 2013; **Jul 11**: 498–505.
17　Morita T, Tsunoda J, Inoue S, *et al.* Terminal sedation for existential distress. *American Journal of Hospice and Palliative Care*. 2000; **17**: 189–95.
18　Ganzini L, Volicer L, Nelson WA, *et al.* Ten myths about decision-making capacity. *Journal of the American Medical Directors Association*. 2005; **6**: S100–4.
19　Castillo LS, Williams BA, Hooper SM, *et al.* Lost in translation: the unintended consequences of advance directive law on clinical care. *Annals of Internal Medicine*. 2011; **154**: 121–8.
20　Sulmasy DP, Snyder L. Substituted interests and best judgments: an integrated model of surrogate decision making. *Journal of the American Medical Association*. 20103; **304**: 1946–7.

21 Glynn SM, Cohen AN, Dixon LB, *et al.* The potential impact of the recovery movement on family interventions for schizophrenia: opportunities and obstacles. *Schizophrenia Bulletin.* 2006; **32**: 451–63.

22 Berk M, Berk L, Udina M, *et al.* Palliative models of care for later stages of mental disorder: maximizing recovery, maintaining hope, and building morale. *Australian & New Zealand Journal of Psychiatry.* 2012; **46**: 92–9.

TO LEARN MORE

- Chochinov HM, Breitbart W, editors. *Handbook of Psychiatry in Palliative Care.* 2nd ed. New York: Oxford University Press; 2012.
- Medical College of Wisconsin. *End of Life/Palliative Care Resource Center Fast Facts.* Available at www.eperc.mcw.edu/EPERC/FastFactsandConcepts (accessed 12 November 2013).
- Nell Ellison. Mental Health Foundation. *Mental Health and Palliative Care Literature Review.* 2008. Available at www.mentalhealth.org.uk/publications/mental-health-palliative-care/ (accessed 12 November 2013).
- National Hospice and Palliative Care Organization. *Ethical Principles: Guidelines for Hospice/ Palliative Care.* Available at www.nhpco.org/ethical-principles (accessed 12 November 2013)
- The Institute for Palliative Medicine at San Diego Hospice. Available at www.palliativemed.org/ Palliative-Care-Psychiatry-Program (accessed 12 November 2013).

TABLE 3.4 Example

Medical indications	*Person preferences*
• Dysphagia and anorexia are symptoms of dementia. • A feeding tube will not prevent aspiration. • Each episode of acute illness the person has suffered has resulted in functional decline.	• An advance directive is present and requests life-sustaining treatment if it would permit or promote reasonable quality of life. • Daughter has power of attorney. • Daughter believes artificial nutrition and hydration should be provided.
Quality of life	*Contextual features*
• Mary's life expectancy based on stage of dementia and symptoms is estimated at six months. • She is no longer able to recognise her children or interact with her grandchildren. • The healthcare professionals at the hospital state she is not actively dying and so treatment should be provided.	• Mary no longer possesses decisional capacity. • There is conflict in the family between Mary and her brothers. • Mary and Eileen are devout Catholics who believe food and water are obligatory even at the end-of-life. • It is legal in the jurisdiction where Mary resides to forego artificial nutrition and hydration, but a higher standard of evidence of the individual's wishes may be required.

CHAPTER 4

Overcoming cultural dilemmas

Geraldine S Pearson

Case Study 4.1 – Jean Phillipe

Jean Phillipe (65), a Haitian male, had a long history of schizophrenia and institution-alisation living in an urban part of the United States. He was experiencing congestive heart failure secondary to a myocardial infarction that went untreated during a period of homelessness. He speaks rarely and his only involved family member is his daughter (45), who visits him regularly in the hospital. He mutters 'I want to die' on a regular basis and his physical health is deteriorating. His daughter would like to bring in a Haitian faith healer from her neighbourhood. Her father does not respond to her questions about this. She is his legal conservator and has initiated Do Not Resuscitate orders (*see* Chapters 3 and 13). Professionals caring for him question what else they could do to make him comfortable. Some are also uncomfortable with the idea of a faith healer coming into the medical unit.

SELF-ASSESSMENT EXERCISE 4.1 – JEAN PHILLIPE (*SEE* ANSWERS ON P. 44)

Time: 20 minutes
1 What are the cultural issues central to the care Jean Phillipe requires on the medical unit where he is hospitalised?
2 How do the professionals on the unit begin to reconcile the cultural influences on Jean Phillipe's care needs and the ways in which they view Jean Phillipe's needs?
3 What can the professionals do to facilitate their own understanding on Jean Phillipe's culture and their response to this?

INTRODUCTION

The concept of culture is an ongoing and essential consideration in all aspects of mental health care. For individuals experiencing historical or current mental health problems, this becomes even more complex and can pose dilemmas to those providing care. Culture, with all its variations and permutations, influences the way individuals and families view their mental health and physical ill-health, how they perceive assessment and treatment, and whether they allow a recommended intervention to occur. Mental health professionals bring all of their own cultural history and personal biases to the interactions.

KEY POINT 4.1

Overcoming the cultural dilemmas presented by those seeking care, whether simple or complex, involves much more than assuming knowledge of a person's cultural background.

It involves knowledge of cultural constructs in self or others that influences therapeutic interventions. This chapter will focus on the cultural dilemmas presented by individuals and their families and the mental health professional's possible reactions to understanding these influences on care.

DEFINITION OF TERMS

Culture, a social and anthropological construct, has been defined by Purnell as:

> the totality of socially transmitted behavioural patterns, arts, beliefs, values, customs, lifeways, and all other products of human work and thought characteristics of a population of people that guide their worldview and decision making.[1]

These beliefs and practices may be conscious or unconscious and tend to be transmitted within the family. Important in this definition is the notion that culture is not homogeneous; knowledge of a culture does not mean the professional understands all the individuals who might fall within that cultural designation.

Populations in the world are constantly migrating and moving.[2] Changes are influenced by the motivator for the move and the transient or permanent nature of the migration. A number of factors will determine the degree of change:

➤ individual
➤ kinship
➤ societal factors.[3]

This makes professionals' acknowledgement of the migration and associated changes in life and cultural identity essential as attempts are made to understand the ethnicity presented by a person. Phinney[4] noted that the norms, values, attitudes and the behaviours that characterise a particular ethnic group may come from a common culture of origin. However, as a population becomes integrated, even partially, in the place where they have migrated, they will, over time and with subsequent generations, take on some of the cultural characteristics of those around them. What emerges is a heterogeneous group of individuals with a variety of cultural influences influencing their functioning and their development of mental health problems. This has far-reaching influences on issues such as perception of mental health, adherence to treatment recommendations, and overcoming barriers to care. Hickling succinctly noted the problem of 'clinical misunderstandings' and recommended the practice of letting individuals self-label ethnic identity and cultural background. He believed this will give a more accurate view of the origin of psychiatric symptoms through 'extensive, empathetic history taking that discounts stereotypical assumptions'.[2] In other words, the professional must maintain an open demeanour when carefully questioning about culture and ethnicity.

SCOPE OF THE PROBLEM

The extensive literature on racial/ethnic discrimination shows that minority populations tend to suffer more from physical ill-health that results in morbidity and mortality. This is multi-determined by factors including:

➤ disproportionate prevalence of less healthy lifestyles
➤ low socioeconomic status
➤ resource-poor neighbourhood environments
➤ poorer access to care.[5]

This is all linked in to cultural barriers to receiving care. Those barriers can include racial discrimination on an interpersonal level and institutional racism within healthcare settings. Gee[6] suggests that discrimination occurs across the gamut of those levels. A lack of cultural understanding of the individual's background and history will contribute to this.

Individuals at all levels are thought to experience cultural dissonance in providing and receiving healthcare. This includes those who provide care and those who receive it.

Case Study 4.2 – Amah

Amah is a child psychiatrist in training whose country of origin, India, is where she received her early education, including medical school. Her care is exemplary and those within her care generally work well with her. Amah speaks English with a slight accent but verbal and written communication skills are excellent. The parents of Julie, a five-year-old girl brought to the mental health clinic for an assessment, are unwilling to continue the care because of Amah's accent. They request a new provider.

SELF-ASSESSMENT EXERCISE 4.2 – AMAH (*SEE* ANSWERS ON P. 44)

Time: 15 minutes

1 What are the cultural issues that might have influenced the request for a new provider?

2 How should the supervisor/manager handle this request and what discussion should occur with the parents prior to deciding on a transition to a new professional?

3 How should the supervisor/manager handle the request for a new clinician with Amah?

While Case Study 4.2 represents a situation where the individuals parenting the child seem to be struggling with the cultural presentation of the professional providing the care, other examples can include the reverse situation. Shavers and others[5] raise the question of unconscious bias in professionals that adversely influences the quality of care given to people of a different culture or race.

> There is also a need to assess how racial/ethnic discrimination faced by racial/ethnic minority health providers within their workplaces (i.e. hospitals and clinics) influences the availability of minority healthcare providers and, as a consequence, minority patient perception of the accessibility of appropriate care.[5]

SELF-ASSESSMENT EXERCISE 4.3 (*SEE* ANSWERS ON P. 45)

Time: 45 minutes

Discuss

1 How do differences in culture influence perceptions of healthcare settings?

2 How do ethnic misunderstandings between professional and person influence quality of care?

3 How can these misunderstandings be acknowledged, interpreted and managed to preserve the therapeutic nature of the care?

Hickling[2] writes about the risks involved in ethnic stereotyping between professionals and those receiving care. He notes that the result can be grave misunderstandings in resulting clinical assessments, leading to potentially inappropriate treatment and increased risk of morbidity and mortality. The example of over-diagnosis of schizophrenia in African-American populations is a result of misunderstanding of cultural paranoia compared to a standard of schizophrenia ill-health.[7]

Core[8] notes that the interface between:

> the cultural frameworks of health-care providers and the cultures of patients and their families is of central importance

... if there is going to be a successful outcome in an intervention that is culturally sensitive.[8]

COLLECTIVIST VERSUS INDIVIDUALISTIC CULTURES[1]

Purnell[9] has identified collectivist versus individualist cultures, and knowledge of this difference can guide the professional working with cultural dilemmas. Individualistic cultures are seen as being *low contexted*, in which ties between groups are loose. People being born into strong cohesive in-groups with extended families that tend to be *highly contexted*, in contrast, characterise collectivist cultures. Examples of highly individualistic cultures are:

- traditional American
- Canadian
- Norwegian
- British
- German
- Swedish cultures.

Examples of collectivist cultures are:

- traditional Arab
- Filipino
- Japanese
- Mexican
- Taiwanese
- Turkish
- Chinese
- Korean
- Latin American
- Native American
- Thai
- Vietnamese.

More world cultures are collectivist than individualist.[1]

Moreover, culture includes many other factors such as lifestyle, gender preferences and spirituality, all influences that must be considered by mental health professionals. The Purnell Model for Cultural Competence (Figure 4.1) illustrates the embedded nature of culturally competent versus culturally incompetent care. Elements of global society, community and family/person interact with a variety of life events. The model identifies primary characteristics of culture as:

- age
- nationality
- colour
- religion.
- generation
- race
- gender

Secondary characteristics of culture include:

- educational status
- occupation
- political beliefs
- enclave identity
- parental status
- sexual orientation
- reason for migration.
- socioeconomic status
- military status
- urban versus rural residence
- marital status
- physical characteristics
- gender issues

The Purnell Model for Cultural Competence

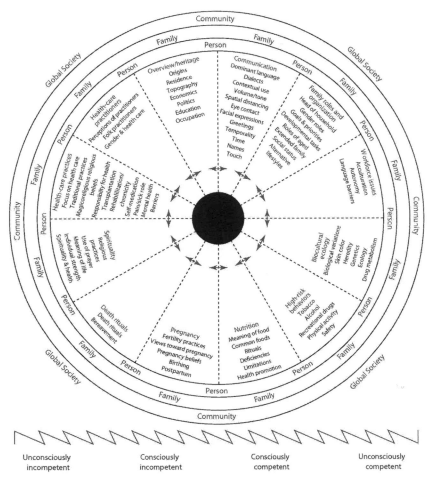

Unconsciously   Consciously   Consciously   Unconsciously
incompetent   incompetent   competent   competent

Primary characteristics of culture: age, generation, nationality, race, color, gender, religion

Secondary characteristics of culture: educational status, socioeconomic status, occupation, military status, political beliefs, urban versus rural residence, enclave identity, marital status, parental status, physical characteristics, sexual orientation, gender issues, and reason for migration (sojourner, immigrant, undocumented status)

Unconsciously incompetent: not being aware that one is lacking knowledge about another culture
Consciously incompetent: being aware that one is lacking knowledge about another culture
Consciously competent: learning about the client's culture, verifying generalizations about the client's culture, and providing culturally specific interventions
Unconsciously competent: automatically providing culturally congruent care to clients of diverse cultures

Model created by Larry D. Purnell, PhD, RN, FAAN. Reprinted with permission.

Figure 4.1 Purnell Model of Cultural Competence
Published in: Purnell L, Paulanka B. *Transcultural Health Care: A Culturally Competent Approach*. Philadelphia: FA Davis; 2008

Purnell further identifies that unconsciously incompetent individuals are not aware that one is lacking knowledge about another culture. In contrast, conscious competence involves learning about the person's culture, verifying generalisations about the person's culture and providing culturally specific interventions. Unconsciously competent individuals automatically provide culturally congruent care to people of diverse cultures.[1] This model has applicability to professionals in all settings and can be used as a guide to inform supervision, consultation and care models.

Case Study 4.3 – Haweeyo

Haweeyo is an immigrant woman from the African nation of Somalia. Aged 45, she speaks little English and has been in Great Britain for two years. When her bizarre behaviour and aggressiveness towards others in a shopping centre results in transport to the emergency room, her extended family quickly gathers in the waiting room and insists on being with her. The professionals in charge of the unit refuse to let the 14 people waiting join her in the small cubicle while the mental health professional conducts an evaluation.

SELF-ASSESSMENT EXERCISE 4.4 – HAWEEYO (*SEE* ANSWERS ON P. 45)

Time: 20 minutes

1 What type of culture does Haweeyo come from?
2 Is the family members' wish to be included in all aspects of the assessment incongruent or congruent with Haweeyo's native culture?
3 How does the mental health professional handle the language barriers inherent in trying to conduct an evaluation?
4 Haweeyo appears malnourished and cachectic. The mental health professional assumes Haweeyo is the victim of forced starvation or abuse. Is this a valid assumption?
5 What actions can the mental health professional take to counter the assumptions being made about Haweeyo?

How does the collectivist versus individualist culture influence the development of cultural dilemmas in care? Purnell noted that in individualist cultures the dominant tenets include:

> individualism, free choice, independence, self-reliance, confidence, doing rather than being, egalitarian relationships, non-hierarchical status, achievement over ascribed status, truth telling, friendliness, openness, futuristic temporality and the ability to control the environment.[1]

In individualist cultures, the individual may be alone when seeking care and may not emphasise a strong, involved family support system. More simply, collectivist societies may focus on 'we-ness' and individualistic notes more emphasis on 'I-ness'.[3,10]

KEY POINT 4.2

In the collectivist culture, the individual will nearly always come with the member(s) of the family and treatment in isolation is not the model to employ. Attempting to separate the person from the family will cause stress. This has to be balanced with the need for privacy and confidentiality for the individual.

The presence of mixed cultures, especially in a family that has acclimated to a new country and culture and has first- and second-generation children and grandchildren who are removed from at least some of the original values by parents and grandparents, can create unique challenges.

Case Study 4.4 – Nayara

Nayara, an educated healthcare professional of Pakistani origins, is living in England with her husband and two adolescent children. Nayara and her husband are devout Muslims and their children hold the same belief. Both boys attend a private secondary school in which their peers are from various nationalities and religious affiliations. When her 16-year-old becomes highly intoxicated and sent to an emergency room for acute alcohol intoxication he is referred to the alcohol services by the attending physician. The physician ascertains that the son has been drinking alcohol on a daily basis for many months and self-identifies with a problem with alcohol use. Nayara refuses this, stating that her son will no longer be attending the school and will be sent to live with relatives in Pakistan. She refuses to discuss this with the psychiatrist and demands that her son be discharged and she be allowed to take him home.

SELF-ASSESSMENT EXERCISE 4.5 – NAYARA (*SEE* ANSWERS ON PP. 45–6)

Time: 30 minutes
1 What is the influence of Pakistani culture and Muslim faith on the parental view of alcohol abuse or addiction in the son?
2 How will you ascertain the discharge plan for this young man if he is allowed to leave the emergency department with his parents?
3 Should the son be allowed to leave the hospital and what information would you need to make this decision?
4 What are the cultural conflicts defining this situation for the:
   • parent
   • son
   • assessing physician?

STEPS TO OVERCOMING CULTURAL DILEMMAS

It is impossible for mental health professionals to know and understand the culture of every person likely to present for care at any given time. Too many cultures and cultural permutations influence healthcare.

KEY POINT 4.3

Professionals need to strive for an attitude of inquiry around the cultural issues presented by people they treat.

This becomes conscious competence or active learning about the person's culture, identifying and clarifying assumptions about that culture and in response, providing mental health interventions that are framed by cultural awareness and sensitivity.

KEY POINT 4.4

In order to be culturally aware and deal with cultural dilemmas, professionals must identify, evaluate and understand their own origins of culture on all levels of their own functioning.

Professionals have to know their own biases and use this knowledge to match their responses to the particular individual or family issues presented in the moment of care. This evaluation must be done continually, like an interpersonal feedback loop, at every stage of evaluation and treatment. Ideally, the individual and family are able to educate the professional on the cultural nuances of their situation. This will only occur if the professional communicates an openness and willingness to hear these issues and has rudimentary knowledge of the cultural issues influencing that particular situation.

Unfortunately, many individuals and families, if they perceive a cultural bias or negative prejudice in the professional, will drop out or end treatment. There are many ways of addressing the professional's differing culture or ethnicity with individuals before an assessment or intervention begins.

KEY POINT 4.5

Acknowledge the differences. Ask the individual and family to help the professional understand and learn about their current culture. This sets a tone of collaboration.

KEY POINT 4.6

When professionals make assumptions, treatment is at risk of sabotage.

CULTURAL DILEMMAS AND INTERVENTION STRATEGIES

What are potential examples of cultural dilemmas that professionals might face? Hickling identifies the:

> dimensionality and complexity in the concepts of ethnicity and culture and in understanding their psychological importance.[2]

Hickling emphasises the need for a careful analysis of the:

> key (interacting) aspects of ethnicity including a person's cultural norms and values; the strength, importance and meaning of ethnic identity; the experiences and attitudes such as powerlessness, discrimination and prejudice that are associated with minority status.[2,4]

This leads to myriad dilemmas that could influence care. Case Studies 4.5–4.8 give brief examples of these.

Case Study 4.5

A man presented to the emergency department of a large metropolitan hospital, accompanied by a police escort. Homeless, he was found hallucinating in front of a large department store and became combative when police attempted to have him leave the site. The professional assigned to triage his care insisted on contacting his extended family even though he denies having any family or familial resources involved in his life.

Cultural dilemma

The professional is from a collectivist culture and although living in an individualist culture currently, continues to believe that it is essential that the family be involved in provision of mental health care.

Cultural intervention

Triage and mental health assessment should be provided to the individual irrespective of the availability of family to support the care. Whilst essential to care, the homeless individual states he has no family support and refuses the information; this must be respected. We must carefully examine our attitudes regarding individuals who refuse to include the family in care.

Case Study 4.6

Insook, an Asian woman (75), a recent immigrant from China, is brought to the office of the primary care clinic in her neighbourhood, appearing as if she is hearing voices and twitching her head and body with involuntary movements. Her son and grandson accompany her to the clinic – both have limited English language skills. When the professional utilised a language service to better understand her complaints and her family's explanation of her issues, they learned that the difficulty was specifically localised to her right ear. An examination revealed that a cockroach was in her ear canal. Once it was extracted, she sat quietly and then fell asleep.

Cultural dilemma

The professional who provided the initial assessment of this person assumed that symptoms were the result of a mental health problem. When native language translation occurred, it showed this to be an entirely different problem, with a physical cause that responded to treatment.

Cultural intervention

A careful health assessment was made of this person, and getting a language service so that all could be understood was the key to ensuring that the real cause of the symptoms was identified and treated. Assumptions were made initially but ruled out before unnecessary mental health interventions were initiated.

Case Study 4.7

Dang, a 63-year-old man who had immigrated to the United States from Vietnam as a 13-year-old, presented in the mental health emergency room with a variety of symptoms. These included depression, suicidal ideation and plan, and poor interpersonal relationships with his wife and children. Unable to work because of his mental health problems, he was admitted to the hospital for the fifth inpatient stay in four years. A review of past records revealed that little assessment had occurred, in previous hospitalisations, around his childhood and adolescent experiences in Saigon. The professional began asking questions about his development and he revealed a strong history of trauma and abuse during his early years that included being left in the city while his family left the country. Intensive psychotherapy began during the hospitalisations and continued at discharge. Dang has not returned to the inpatient unit in nearly two years and remains in treatment.

Cultural dilemma

A careful developmental history of this individual's past life experiences in Vietnam as a child and young adolescent might have helped identify the early origins of his current mental health problem. When the mental health professional carefully assessed history and realised where he had been born, speculating on traumatic life experiences, the individual was able to identify his early deprivation, separation from family and loss of identity as he immigrated to another country.

Cultural intervention

While a careful developmental history of all individuals is warranted regardless of their age, it is difficult to do this on a busy inpatient unit with a short length of stay and limited time for history gathering. With this individual, it was essential that the professional understand his background as a child in war-torn Saigon in the 1960s–1970s historical period. Once the professional discovered that his family had left him behind in the country and he made his way, alone, to a refugee camp, the roots of his depression and isolation were better understood.

Case Study 4.8

Jose, a Latino male (17), presents to the mental health clinic with symptoms of depression and anxiety. He speaks of being a transgender individual and beginning this year living as a woman, in preparation for his eventual gender reassignment surgery. While he initially states that his family is supportive, he also admits that they are confused by his behaviour and might accept that he could be homosexual, but have no understanding of the complexities of being transgender. He is adamantly opposed to including them in his treatment. The professional, also Latino, states to his supervisor that he believes Jose is making a mistake in choosing this surgery.

Cultural dilemma

The young man is caught by the cultural dissonance of his decision with his family who do not understand why he wishes to change his gender. He is also confronted with the unconscious and conscious beliefs and attitudes of the culturally similar professional who is providing assessment and treatment in the clinic. Jose is at risk of feeling unsupported and unheard in the therapeutic assessment and intervention.

Cultural intervention

The professional is advised to obtain supervision or consultation on the conscious and unconscious ways his own cultural background as a Latino male affects the way he deals with this individual. Once that occurs he will be able to help the young man sort through the issues influencing his depression, his sense of himself, his involvement of his family and the life decisions he is making.

HELPFUL INTERVENTIONS IN OVERCOMING CULTURAL DILEMMAS

There are significant pressures for provision of mental health care. Limited numbers of professionals from all disciplines are available to treat an expanding population of individuals requiring care. This worldwide need for mental health services makes taking the time to define and understand the influences of culture on practice more challenging. This, coupled with the complexity of migrating cultures and the resulting heterogeneity of various family members, requires time, patience and curiosity to identify influences on the mental health care and then carefully plan culturally focused treatment.

Traditional psychotherapy that is based on culturally adapted interventions for individuals, families and groups should be modified to match the person's cultural context.[2]

KEY POINT 4.7

The professional providing the treatment must carefully and rigorously understand his or her cultural background and ethnic influences on the style of treatment provided.

KEY POINT 4.8

Models of supervision and peer review are excellent arenas for dealing with this.

Professionals may choose not to work with particular groups of people if they are unable to reconcile their own culture with issues presented by the individuals they see. Acknowledgement of this is preferable to biased interventions that may result in individuals leaving treatment precipitously.

It is essential that education and training for professionals contains a strong core of cultural education and awareness training that endures through the educational process. Core[8] suggested four educational strategies for educating professionals.

1 **Knowledge-oriented strategies** – Providing the student with the basic knowledge about their own and other cultures.
2 **Awareness-oriented strategies** – Emphasising experiential processes and a focus on the student's ability to see situations from their own and others' viewpoint with accuracy.
3 **Affect-oriented strategies** – Focusing on the emotions involved when dealing with value-laden diversity issues.
4 **Skill-oriented strategies** – Striving to nurture the student's ability to perform effectively in multicultural interactions.[8]

Models of care have to focus on all stages of the treatment process. Gore[8] suggested the idea of cultural mentoring of new healthcare professionals to further their understanding of the cultural context of their work. Certainly, during treatment it is essential that the professional gently queries the individual and family about their health practices and beliefs and makes this an ongoing aspect of care.

KEY POINT 4.9

Follow-up services should be individualised to the needs of the person receiving care, considering cultural background and biases.

CONCLUSIONS

Recognising, understanding and intervening in cultural dilemmas presented during clinical interactions with individuals and families requires a continual air of inquiry on the part of professionals. It is impossible to have complete knowledge or understanding of the multitude of cultures that can potentially present for medical or mental health care. The following are realistic ways of dealing with cultural dilemmas.

KEY POINT 4.10

- Foster an atmosphere of institutional cultural sensitivity, especially in geographic areas where the professionals are generally not of the same ethnicity or culture as the individuals requesting care.
- Ensure that educational materials are available to teach professionals about cultural differences in the populations they are treating.
- Enhance performance with regular supervision that assists professionals in understanding their own unconscious biases that may adversely influence care delivery.
- Encourage an air of inquiry around cultural dilemmas; asking individuals and families seeking care to assist in understanding their family rules and culture.

It takes work, effort, and commitment to address and overcome cultural dilemmas. It is essential that these efforts occur to narrow the existing cultural divide between many professionals providing care and the people they treat.

ACKNOWLEDGEMENT

The author and editors are grateful to Professor Larry Purnell for permitting the use of his model for cultural competence (Figure 4.1).

REFERENCES

1 Purnell LD. Application of transcultural theory to practice: The Purnell Model. In: Cooper DB, Cooper J, editors. *Palliative Care within Mental Health: principles and philosophy*. London: Radcliffe Publishing; 2013. pp. 22–44.
2 Hickling FW. Understanding patients in multicultural settings: a personal reflection on ethnicity and culture in clinical practice. *Ethnicity & Health*. 2012; **17**: 203–16.
3 Bhugra D. Cultural identities and cultural congruency: a new model for evaluating mental distress in immigrants. *Acta Psychiatrica Scandinavica*. 2005; **111**: 84–93.
4 Phinney J. When we talk about American ethnic groups, what do we mean? *American Psychologist*. 1996; **51**: 918–27.
5 Shavers VL, Fagan P, Jones D, et al. The state of research on racial/ethnic discrimination in the receipt of health care. *American Journal of Public Health*. 2012; **102**: 953–66.
6 Gee GC. A multilevel analysis of the relationship between institutional and individual racial discrimination and health status. *American Journal of Public Health*. 2008; **98**(9 Suppl.): S48–S56.
7 Whaley AL, Geller PA. Toward a cognitive process model of ethnic/racial biases in clinical judgment. *Review of General Psychology*. 2007; **11**: 75–96.
8 Core L. Treatment across cultures: is there a model? *International Journal of Therapy and Rehabilitation*. 2008; **15**: 519–27.

9 Purnell L. *Guide to Culturally Competent Care*. Philadelphia: FA Davis; 2009.
10 Hofstede G. *Culture's Consequences: abridged*. Beverly Hills, CA: Sage; 1984.

TO LEARN MORE

• Purnell L. Application to transcultural theory to practice: the Purnell Model. In: Cooper DB, Cooper J, editors. *Palliative Care within Mental Health: principles and philosophy*. London/New York: Radcliffe Publishing; 2012. Chapter 3, pp. 22–44.

ANSWERS TO SELF-ASSESSMENT EXERCISE 4.1 – JEAN PHILLIPE (*SEE* P. 30)

1 The cultural issues presenting in this case study are the individual's Haitian culture and the way this influences his perception of his ill-health and hospitalisation. His daughter's culture, her belief in a faith healer and her views on death and dying are operative. In addition, mental health issues influences may have contributed to his homelessness.

2 The professionals reconcile the identified differences through frequent conversations with each other, unit leadership, this individual and his daughter. They work to understand the concept of the Haitian faith healer, and the daughter is pushing for an intervention her father does not support. They identify the changes in his care needs as his medical condition worsens.

3 Professionals can seek consultation about Haitian culture, read, speak to the man's daughter, and better understand how this has influenced his life.

ANSWERS TO SELF-ASSESSMENT EXERCISE 4.2 – AMAH (*SEE* P. 33)

1 The cultural differences between the individual and family receiving care and the physician providing care are obvious given the provider's accent. The family has made assumptions about the provision of care not being 'good enough' and they hint that the provider cannot understand their issues. The predominant cultural issues are likely around ethnicity, race and language.

2 The clinic should follow the protocol established to deal with individuals who request a different professional. Interventions should occur with the family requesting different care and with the physician attempting to provide the care. While the family requires support, a gentle intervention exploring their concerns might assist them in trusting a new psychiatrist. It is possible that culture is not the only issue they are worried about. Other concerns might involve stigma, the role of medication in treatment and the process of psychiatric diagnosis.

3 These misunderstandings must be handled with care, sensitivity and attention to the involved individuals. Hopefully it becomes a teaching moment for all, around the role culture plays in trusting a mental health professional and for ascertaining the ambivalence the family might have in mental health treatment provided by any individual, regardless of culture.

ANSWERS TO SELF-ASSESSMENT EXERCISE 4.3 (*SEE* P. 33)

Possible answers for the discussion

1   Culture is the basis for perceptions of healthcare practices. It is linked to illness/wellness, origins of illness, spiritual beliefs and healing practices that are culturally based.

2   These misunderstandings, if not resolved, can cause healthcare relationships to end precipitously, resulting in poorer health and lack of treatment. Care only has quality if it can occur in a mutually agreeable manner with the goal of improved functioning and resolution of the crisis that caused the illness state.

3   The best way to acknowledge misunderstandings is to speak of them, analyse them in supervision relationships, self-correct and attempt to preserve the care relationship with an air of openness and curiosity.

ANSWERS TO SELF-ASSESSMENT EXERCISE 4.4 – HAWEEYO (*SEE* P. 36)

---

1   A Somalian culture is likely a collectivist, family-centred culture in which members of the community care for each other.

2   This wish is completely congruent with a collectivist culture.

3   There are many ways to handle a language difference. Using a community translator, translator services in the care setting or a trusted family friend or family member, at least for the short term, might be useful. There are programs that run on cell phones that can assist in translation.

4   This is *not* a valid assumption. This individual might be physically ill, might be struggling with parasitic disease, or having difficulty acclimating to the food available to her. All of these issues need to be explored.

5   The provider can take a leadership role in identifying concerns about this woman and her physical status, urging caution in making judgements. The provider can also point out the cultural issues that might influence her physical status.

ANSWERS TO SELF-ASSESSMENT EXERCISE 4.5 – NAYARA (*SEE* P. 37)

---

1   Use of alcohol or other drugs is strictly forbidden in the Muslim faith. The conservative Pakistani cultural background of the woman also forbids use of substances. This is creating dissonance between belief system and actual issues presented by Nayara's son.

2   The answer to this question depends on the level of acuity in the clinical presentation of this young man. His level of danger to self must be carefully assessed.

3   It is unclear whether he should be allowed to leave the hospital with his parents. Again, his level of danger to self and others will likely influence the decisions made by professionals. Psychoeducation must be attempted with the parents, even though their cultural beliefs are making acceptance of their son's alcoholism

extremely difficult, if not impossible. Other community supports or family members might be enlisted to help with this.

4 The parents are finding the social situations their son has been experiencing dissonant with their cultural and religious beliefs. It would be important to ascertain how much of the behaviour is related to experimentation versus more serious and long-term substance use. The physician assessing the individual must ascertain his views about returning home and then going to Pakistan. Care and assessment must proceed carefully.

CHAPTER 5

The family

Robin Davidson, Tracy Anderson

INTRODUCTION

KEY POINT 5.1

A family can provide emotional warmth, responsiveness and stability. These characteristics can be just as important for a grandparent at the end-of-life as the newborn baby at life's beginning.

The family is the elementary unit of organisation in the lives of human beings across most cultures. So-called strong family resilience can, in itself, help people cope with crisis situations and promote positive mental health. Alternatively, families with high levels of expressed emotion can promote psychopathology. Dysfunctional family dynamics have been identified as making an aetiological contribution to almost all mental health problems, from chronic schizophrenia to transient situational anxiety.

Contemporary understanding of the family originates from systems theory. This identifies family members as parts of a system in which there are numerous interactions, all of which contribute to its maintenance. This approach has in turn led to the development of a range of systemic family therapies, which have been popular for almost 50 years. Family research has, by and large, focused on developmental disorders of the young. There has been less research on what constitutes resilience in families facing the death of a loved one. In this chapter we present several familiar scenarios faced by families and professionals working in mental health and palliative care settings.

The chapter is a guide and potentially challenging issues are highlighted using practical examples. If the reaction of family members before and during the death of a relative is poorly handled, it can lead to long-term feelings of guilt, dysthymia (a form of chronic depression), anxiety or anger. Here we apply the principles and philosophy of palliative care to long-term mental health but are primarily focusing on end-of-life. We believe this is a pivotal time when poorly managed family conflict and confusion may have particular long-term psychological sequelae.

There are some pre-loss family variables, which predict complicated post-loss mental health problems.[1] These can include:

➤ marital quality
➤ attachment style
➤ premorbid depression
➤ caregiver burden
➤ pessimistic life orientation.

The latter is regarded as increasingly useful when trying to get an idea of the risk of psychological morbidity among family members dealing with death and dying. Dispositional pessimism and optimism can be assessed using the Life Orientation Test, which would seem to have better predictive validity than more general personality measures.[2] Mental health professionals who work with family members, particularly those who act as caregivers, should pay particular attention to these predictors if they are to guard against longer-term mental health problems associated with the eventual loss of a loved one.

KEY POINT 5.2

Sensitive, appropriate, evidence-based family involvement is important in palliative care settings.

Despite the above, professionals sometimes report that they feel too busy to speak with the family or may even resent the fact that family discussions can take longer than their actual interaction with the person who is ill. It is important for the future well-being of family members that the correct balance is struck. The family can provide important insights about their relative's life, interests and previously expressed wishes. Family members can help each person to communicate with professionals and indeed can often facilitate their relative being cared for in a preferred location rather than necessarily being admitted to hospital (*see* Chapter 6).[3]

To be a primary carer for a relative at the end-of-life, be that a parent, partner, child or sibling, can be stressful for many reasons, and if not approached appropriately by professionals may have permanent mental health implications. This relationship between very poor communication by a professional and long-term mental health problems is illustrated in Case Study 5.6. Some sources of stress are summarised in Box 5.1. The NICE guidelines[4] highlight the need for appropriate, tailored and timely support for family carers. This is not only enabling for the family member but is also in the best interests of their ill relative, who may be more concerned about the future well-being of the family than they are about themselves.

SELF-ASSESSMENT EXERCISE 5.1

Time: 10 minutes
- Consider some of the potential sources of stress encountered by the family at the end-of-life.
- Compare your thoughts and feeling with those listed in Box 5.1.

BOX 5.1 Sources of family end-of-life stress

- Sadness about impending loss of a loved one.
- Anger about delay in diagnosis or lack of effectiveness of treatment.
- Anxiety about the symptoms the person will experience and how they will be managed.
- Responsibility for being involved in treatment decisions.
- The challenge of supporting a family member emotionally throughout a difficult time.
- The difficulty associated with providing the practical daily care for an ill relative.
- Guilt, if unable to provide that care at home.
- Responsibility for sharing difficult information with other family members, including children.
- Regret or guilt about previous issues in the relationship.
- Financial concerns.

TAILORED, TIMELY AND EFFECTIVE FAMILY SUPPORT

It is important to promote a sense of family efficacy.

KEY POINT 5.3

Family members should, if they and the person wish, be involved routinely in the care of their relative and be assured that their experience and views are valued.

The family should be afforded timely updates on their relative's progress. This symbiotic relationship can be enabling for both family members and professionals. The family will feel involved and will be aware of what is likely to happen as the ill-health progresses. Alternatively, professionals can routinely gain further information about how the person's symptoms were prior to admission, previous coping strategies, and any recent deterioration and how quickly this has happened. It is good practice to have the family present when sharing bad news and to keep them informed regarding results of investigations and future management plans. If the ill relative expresses the wish for information without family present, this of course must be respected.

COMMUNICATION AND THERAPY

It is important to take time with family members and allow space for appropriate emotional expression. Often a professional, through the simple use of reflective listening, can facilitate this. Sometimes family members will need more formal support to help them work through painful emotions and thoughts. Cognitive behavioural therapy (CBT), tailored for use in palliative care, is an example of one such supportive therapy (*see* Case Study 5.1). Early CBT intervention can be provided by any professional with the appropriate brief training in CBT. Clearly, if more specialised intervention is required, referral of the family to counselling or the Clinical Psychology team may be necessary. However, there is now good evidence that nursing staff with brief training, of a matter of hours, in palliative CBT techniques are particularly helpful to people with life-limiting ill-health and their families.[5]

Case Study 5.1 – Barbara – Part I

Barbara's mother has just been admitted for hospice care. She has been deteriorating recently and needed increasing support at home. Barbara, who is unmarried, moved in with her mother several months before and was looking after her 24 hours a day with little additional family support. Barbara was getting very little sleep, was struggling to cope and was getting easily frustrated with her mother. Barbara has now almost moved into the hospice, where nurses are trying to encourage her to go home and get some rest. She is not keen to do so and is expressing increasingly depressive ideation. A professional is having CBT structured conversations with Barbara and through careful and sensitive questioning ascertains that she feels guilty because she promised her mother that she would not let her be admitted to a hospice but would care for her in a treasured home environment. Moreover, Barbara feels angry with herself and regrets getting frustrated, because they have always had a good relationship. Barbara does not want this to change in her mother's final weeks. The only way to attenuate her guilt is to be with her mother as much as possible and support her in the same way as she did at home.

In this scenario some specific thoughts, feelings and behaviours can be identified and linked together: The *feelings* are guilt, regret, self-annoyance and frustration. The *cognitions* include:
1 I have let my mother down by not keeping my promise
2 I cannot cope
3 I am completely ruining my wonderful relationship with her
4 I cannot leave her here alone.

These feelings and cognitions combine to produce the ultimately dysfunctional *behaviour*, i.e. not leaving the hospice and self-neglect.

Case Study 5.1 – Barbara – Part II

The professional, who had completed a brief course in palliative CBT care, was able to recognise the negative thoughts and systematically but caringly challenge them as follows:

1 Thought – I have let my mother down by not keeping my promise.
   Challenge
   - When you think logically about how you have cared for your mother recently, do you think you have let her down?
   - How would your mother view it?
   - If you were talking to a friend in a similar situation, how would you view it?
   - What have the professionals been saying? That it was important your mother came to the hospice for reassessment because her condition has deteriorated so rapidly it is important to see if there is any cause of this that may be reversible.

2 Thought – I cannot cope any more, I've nothing left.
   Challenge
   - This is a realistic thought because in the current situation you cannot cope, but hospice professionals are hopeful that your mother's condition may improve and will provide extra care at home. This may improve your ability to cope.

3 Thought – I am ruining my good relationship with Mum.
   Challenge
   - Frustration in this situation is completely normal. Exhaustion is likely to be contributing, therefore if you get more support and rest you are likely to be able to cope better.

4 Thought – I cannot leave her here alone.
   Challenge
   - Is she alone? What is your knowledge of how responsive the hospice professionals are to her needs and how they care for her?
   - If she is discharged home, you will be the main carer again and will fulfil that role much better if you have taken the opportunity of a good break.
   - It is likely that a priority for your mother is that you are looked after too.

When thoughts are identified and challenged this often helps deal with negative feelings. Some simple behavioural goals can be agreed upon, for example going out for an hour for a cup of coffee knowing that a professional will phone if necessary. Hopefully this will provide reassurance that Barbara's mother is well looked after. This can be gradually increased to an overnight at home, and Barbara will see that this is benefiting her, and subsequently will benefit her mother.

Cognitive behavioural therapy (CBT) is only one of several family therapy interventions that have been developed in general mental health populations but which can be extrapolated to support families in palliative care. The advice given to Barbara may seem simple common sense, but health professionals report that a basic knowledge of CBT can be empowering and help add structure to day-to-day, difficult conversations.[5]

> **KEY POINT 5.4**
>
> Whatever the therapy, it should be delivered with warmth and sensitivity.

It is these so-called therapies or 'non-specific variables' which can account for greater positive outcome variance than even the psychotherapeutic 'techniques' employed. In establishing the optimum therapeutic alliance with a family member, the overarching priority is good communication skills (*see* Chapter 15). The person and their family want to feel listened to and respected. If the individual consents, it is important that information is honestly shared with their family. Difficult conversations should be framed in a way that the family will easily understand and they should be conducted in a private and uninterrupted location. It is good practice to involve other members of the intra-/inter-disciplinary team, who may be providing ongoing support for the family. Families may feel overwhelmed with the information, so it is important to keep checking that each understands and that they want the conversation to continue. They may need some time to reflect and the opportunity to come back with further questions at another time.

The breaking bad news guidelines, although initially produced to guide discussion with the individual, can also be useful when professionals are relating to families.[6] Breaking bad news badly can produce secondary trauma and occasionally result in post-traumatic stress symptoms, as illustrated in Case Study 5.6.

DIFFICULT FAMILY ISSUES

There are a number of common, but potentially challenging, situations that professionals can face when working with families in palliative care settings. Some typical examples are listed in Box 5.2.

SELF-ASSESSMENT EXERCISE 5.2

> **Time: 15 minutes**
> - Consider your own working environment. What difficulties have you experienced or witnessed other professionals experiencing in terms of family conflict?

BOX 5.2 Common family presentations

> - Family disagrees with the wishes of the individual.
> - Disagreement between family members about the care of their family.
> - Family unhappy about decisions made by professionals.
> - Family requests that their relative is not told diagnosis or prognosis.
> - Family asking for information without the consent of their relative.

There is no clear single answer to these conflicts, but each requires a sensitive and thoughtful approach. While some of the situations can be resolved quickly, non-resolution can, as noted above, have long-term adverse psychological consequences. There are a number of end-of-life situations in which conflict is particularly likely between professionals and families of people with life-limiting ill-health, and indeed can lead at times to intra-family disputes. The following examples cover some common situations of potential conflict and misunderstanding. We have tried through the use of case studies to demonstrate how health professionals can minimise the possibility of initial conflict and protracted distress.

The lack of capacity

In a situation when someone lacks capacity to make medical decisions, a careful judgement must be made about what treatment is in the person's best interest. Any such decision should take into account the person's previously stated wishes or beliefs and family preferences. Treatment should only be provided if considered to be of net benefit.[3] If this is uncertain, it is reasonable to start the treatment and regularly review and stop if there is no improvement. What is important is that families do not feel that they are responsible for making decisions on behalf of their relative, as this can add to already existing perceived burden. The family members need to understand that their views and their knowledge of what the individual's views might be are important, but that the responsibility for the decision lies with the intra-disciplinary team.[3] For a person to have capacity to make a decision regarding their treatment they must be able to:

➤ understand and retain the relevant information
➤ believe the information
➤ weigh up the information
➤ arrive at a choice
➤ communicate that choice.

It is assumed that each individual has capacity unless proven otherwise. An individual can have capacity for some decisions but not others, and should be empowered to make as many decisions for her- or himself as possible. Any reversible cause for impaired capacity should be considered and every effort should be made to maximise capacity.

KEY POINT 5.5

In the interests of confidentiality, professionals must obtain permission from the person to share details of their ill-health with family members.

If the person is unable to communicate, it is reasonable to assume that he or she would want family members to be given information, unless previously stated otherwise.[3]

Cardiopulmonary resuscitation (CPR) for people with advanced ill-health

For individuals with advanced ill-health whose condition is deteriorating and death is expected in the near future, CPR is very unlikely to be successful.

KEY POINT 5.6

Even if CPR is successful in restarting the heart it may not prolong life, but instead prolong the dying process, resulting in death being traumatic and undignified.

In the above situation, a decision should be made and recorded that CPR should not be attempted. If there is a possibility that CPR may be successful and the person has capacity, it is appropriate to discuss the benefits and burdens with that person and seek his or her opinion. It is of central importance to ensure families are aware of the reasons behind a decision not to attempt CPR,[3,7] as this is a frequent and significant source of distress among family members.

Advance care planning

Advance care planning is a process of discussion between a person and an appropriately trained professional about their future care and treatment. It is made when a person has capacity and comes into effect when capacity is lost. It can involve decisions regarding specific treatments that would be delivered in specific circumstances, for example:

➤ fluids
➤ artificial nutrition
➤ antibiotics
➤ resuscitation.

It can include preferences about where the person would like to be cared for at the end-of-life, if and when they lose capacity. It is good practice to involve family members in these discussions with the person's consent, to minimise any future disagreement. Advance care planning differs from an Advance Decision to Refuse Treatment (ADRT) because it is not a legal document but is a useful guide to what ill relatives would want in a particular circumstance. The individual and family should be made aware that any views expressed will be considered but that there is no guarantee their wishes can be carried out as it will depend on the specific situation.[3,8,9] The following case studies are fairly common and illustrate these issues.

Case Study 5.2 – Avril

Avril made an advance care plan stating that when she became unresponsive she did not want to be admitted to hospital or treated with antibiotics or resuscitation attempted. One family member who was present when the ACP was completed is in full agreement with this. Another daughter, who lives abroad, disagrees and insists that her mother is admitted to hospital for active treatment.

SELF-ASSESSMENT EXERCISE 5.3 (*SEE* ANSWERS ON P. 59)

Time: 10 minutes

1   What are the main issues to remember regarding advance care plans?
2   What is the appropriate thing to do in this situation?

Case Study 5.3 – Dennis

Dennis (85) had previously and definitely stated to his family that he would like to die at home and his family want to fulfil his wishes. However, he is in a lot of distress because of pain. His family are exhausted, stressed and do not feel able to manage him at home.

SELF-ASSESSMENT EXERCISE 5.4 (*SEE* ANSWERS ON P. 60)

Time: 10 minutes

• What discussion would you have with his family?

Withholding information

Any person has the right to receive information about their diagnosis, prognosis and treatment options. They also have the right to refuse any information regarding their ill-health. Families often want to protect the relative with life-limiting ill-health from the stress of knowing the diagnosis. It is not appropriate for a family to demand that information is not shared, especially if that information is necessary to enable the person to make an informed decision about investigations or treatment.[3,9]

Case Study 5.4 – Angelina

Angelina (56) has a recent diagnosis of early dementia and has also been diagnosed with lung cancer. The whole family are in full agreement that they do not want Angelina to be told she has cancer.

SELF-ASSESSMENT EXERCISE 5.5 (*SEE* ANSWERS ON P. 60)

Time: 10 minutes

1   What issues need to be considered?
2   What is the appropriate approach?

Artificial hydration at the end-of-life

Hydration is a very sensitive issue and it is common for families to think that their relative will die a distressing death without artificial hydration, so it is important to discuss the withdrawal of fluids with families before it happens. This can often cause great distress among family members. Every effort must be made to ensure family members understand their relative will not suffer as a result.

KEY POINT 5.7

It is useful for the family to be told that the sensation of thirst decreases at the end-of-life and good mouth care can alleviate dry mouth as effectively as intravenous (IV) fluids.

Intravenous fluids are a medical treatment and the benefits and burdens of these as well as other treatments need to be weighed up at the end-of-life. There are times – unless the person is dying – when it may be appropriate to continue fluids, for example to minimise opioid side effects in a person with renal failure or in a person with bowel obstruction who is unable to take any oral intake because of the risk of vomiting.

KEY POINT 5.8

Giving IV fluids to a person who is dying can also have adverse effects; for example, fluid overload, chest secretions and oedema.[8]

There has been considerable debate in the literature about stopping fluids inappropriately.[9] They should only be stopped if there is agreement that the person is dying. If there is any chance that the person's condition may improve, fluids may be continued unless causing harm. This must be reviewed by the intra-disciplinary team regularly. Family anxiety about stopping fluids in a setting where they are not causing harm to their relative may be a reason to continue in the short term while discussing the situation with family and helping them accept prognosis.

Case Study 5.5 – Lucy

Lucy (90), a grandmother, is in the terminal phase of ill-health and unresponsive with no oral intake. The medical team feel she is in the last days of life and have withdrawn all active treatments. Her family arrive and see that intravenous fluids have been stopped and are upset that Lucy is going to 'die of dehydration'.

SELF-ASSESSMENT EXERCISE 5.6 (*SEE* ANSWERS ON PP. 60–1)

Time: 10 minutes
- What issues would you discuss with the family?

Many families fear that the last moments will be filled with distress. This is infrequent and so it is critically important to share with the family that it is most likely their relative will not be distressed but will become increasingly drowsy and less responsive, breathing may become erratic with longer periods between breaths, before the heart and lungs stop completely. This awareness can be comforting for family members and to some extent attenuate their apprehension.

PROTECTION OF MENTAL HEALTH

The different areas highlighted above have a number of common components. It is essential for professionals to be sensitive to the needs, questions and concerns of family members. Information must be tailored to where the family is in relation to the psychological and physical ill-health trajectory of their relative. If this contact between family and healthcare professionals is not predicated on the basic counselling principles of empathy, congruence and unconditional regard, then, as noted above, it can have far-reaching consequences for the family member's mental state. Anne's story (*see* Case Study 5.6) highlights the risks in this regard.

Case Study 5.6 – Anne

Anne went to the hospital with her husband Tom. They had attended the 'out patients' clinic for test results and it was there and then agreed that Tom should be admitted. Anne was asked to speak to the registrar in one of the rather busy waiting rooms. She had been made aware by the general practitioner/medical doctor that Tom possibly had cancer, but at that stage she knew little more. After introducing himself and saying a few words which she has since forgotten, the doctor stated, 'it is nearly the end of the line for your husband'. A year later, sadly, Tom died.

It is now two years since his death and it is that brief encounter which still causes Anne great distress. One of the criteria for defining trauma is sudden awareness of existential threat. Anne continues to describe daytime intrusions about the conversation with the registrar, a startle response, emotional numbing, lack of motivation and avoidance behaviour. This encounter was a more significant aetiological trigger of her post-traumatic stress disorder (PTSD) than the actual death of her husband.

Of course we cannot protect everyone from possible long-term mental health problems, which can be triggered by a relative's ill-health and death.

KEY POINT 5.9

There is no doubt that sensitive care from professionals is important in helping the family experience a 'good death' and thus, at least to some extent, affording protection from adverse psychological effects.

There is no doubt that traumatic circumstances surrounding the death of a relative can be significant in the development of later depression, addictive behaviours, pathological grief, generalised anxiety adjustment disorders and, surprisingly, in individuals who may be already vulnerable, i.e. long-term agoraphobia. It is salutary that a key literature review of this area has found a prevalence of mental health problems in carers and family of relatives with life-limiting ill-health to be between 20% and 30%.[10] Recent work with bereaved family members has indicated that what were called 'environmental comfort', 'physical and psychological comfort', 'being respected as an individual' and 'appropriate opioid treatment' contributed to the evaluation of a 'good death'.

KEY POINT 5.10

It has been found that prolonged and aggressive treatment in the final weeks were perceived by family as barriers to the attainment of a good death.[11]

FINAL CONTACT

Families often need some guidance about communicating with ill relatives and can find it difficult to share their emotions honestly as they want to protect each other. Family members often have the difficult job of communicating bad news to other family members, including children. Support and evidence-based guidance can help prepare them for these difficult conversations.

There are other more specific emotional demands which families face when coping with the death of a relative. The intensity of these particular stressors will depend on a whole range of variables like the age of the dying relative, emotional closeness, gender, historical relationship, attachment representation, personality, length of ill-health and degree of long-term disability.[12] Clearly, for example, there are specific issues for families who face the loss of a child, and indeed psychological distress experienced by children arising from parental/sibling ill-health and death.

CONCLUSION

In this chapter we have essentially concentrated on producing guidance for frontline health professionals who are helping families cope with the death of a close, adult relative. This is of central importance not only in promoting familial resilience before and after a relative's death but also in reducing the possibility of longer-term mental health problems.

REFERENCES

1 Tomarken A, Holland J, Schacter S, *et al*. Factors of complicated grief pre-death in caregivers of cancer patients. *Psycho-Oncology*. 2008; **17**: 105–11.
2 Robinson-Whelen S, Kim C, MacCallum R, *et al*. Distinguishing optimism from pessimism in older adults. *Journal of Personality and Social Psychology*. 1997; **73**: 1345–53.

3 General Medical Council: *Treatment and Care towards the End of Life: good practice in decision making*. London: General Medical Council; 2010. Available at: www.gmc-uk.org/End_of_life.pdf_32486688.pdf (accessed 15 January 2014).

4 National Institute for Health and Clinical Excellence. *Improving Supportive and Palliative Care for Adults with Cancer*. London: National Institute for Health and Clinical Excellence; 2004. Available at: www.nice.org.uk/csgsp (accessed 15 January 2014).

5 Anderson T, Watson M, Davidson R. The use of cognitive behavioural therapy techniques for anxiety and depression in hospice patients: a feasibility study. *Palliative Medicine*. 2008; **22**: 814–21.

6 National Council for Hospice and Specialist Palliative Care Services. *Breaking Bad News ... Regional Guidelines*. London: National Council for Hospice and Specialist Palliative Care Services; 2003. Available at: www.dhsspsni.gov.uk/breaking_bad_news.pdf (accessed 15 January 2014).

7 Resuscitation Council (UK). *Resuscitation Guidelines*. London: Resuscitation Council; 2010. Available at: www.resus.org.uk/pages/guide.htm (accessed 15 January 2014).

8 Watson M, Lucas C, Hoy A, *et al. Palliative Adult Network Guidelines*. 3rd ed. London: Royal College of General Practitioners, Northern Ireland Cancer Network, NHS Network; 2011.

9 General Medical Council. *Consent: patients and doctors making decisions together*. London: General Medical Council; 2008. Available at: www.gmc-uk.org/static/documents/content/Consent_-_English_0911.pdf (accessed 15 January 2014).

10 Pitceathly C, Maguire P. The psychological impact of cancer on patients partners, partners and other key relatives: a review. *European Journal of Cancer*. 2003; **39**: 1517–24.

11 Mitsunori M, Tatsuya M, Kasuki S, *et al*. Factors contributing to evaluation of a good death from the bereaved family member's perspective. *Psycho-Oncology*. 2008; **17**: 612–20.

12 Nijboer C, Triemstra M, Tempelaar R, *et al*. Determinants of caregiving experience and mental health of partners on cancer patients. *Cancer*. 1999; **9**: 232–42.

13 Department of Health. *More Care, Less Pathway: a review of the Liverpool Care Pathway*. London: Department of Health; 2013. Available at: www.gov.uk/government/uploads/system/uploads/attachment_data/file/212450/Liverpool_Care_Pathway.pdf (accessed 15 January 2014).

TO LEARN MORE

- Stedeford A. *Facing Death: patients, families and professionals*. 2nd ed. Oxfordshire: Sobell Publications; 1994.
- Redgrove M, Smyth A. Hearing the pain of the carer. In: Cooper J, editor. *Stepping into Palliative Care 2: care and practice*. 2nd ed. Oxford/Seattle: Radcliffe Medical Press; 2006. pp. 181–8.
- Sadler A. Caring for the family. In: Cooper DB, editor. *Care in Mental Health–Substance Use*. London: Radcliffe Publishing; 2011. pp. 31–40.

ANSWERS TO SELF-ASSESSMENT EXERCISE 5.3 (*SEE* P. 55)

---

1 An ACP is a useful guide to an individual's wishes, but is not a legal document. The statement on the ACP must be applicable to the current situation. The best interests of the ill relative must be the priority.

2 It is appropriate to fulfil the person's previously stated wishes even if some of the family disagree, but this needs to be sensitively discussed to minimise conflict. If there is continued disagreement, it is appropriate to seek a second opinion regarding the assessment in the best interests of their relative.

ANSWERS TO SELF-ASSESSMENT EXERCISE 5.4 (*SEE* P. 55)

- Listen to their concerns and appreciate that their guilt is valid, but focus on working together to achieve what is best for Dennis. Being in the place he desires, but having uncontrolled symptoms, cannot be appropriate and would be unlikely to be their father's current wish if he was able to state it. When Dennis made a decision about place of care he could not have predicted the exact circumstances and implications of carrying out his wishes. Reassure the family that they are not letting him down – they are making a positive decision about what is best for him and for them. Furthermore, reassure them that their key role is to make the most of the last days with him and it may be easier to do this in a hospital or hospice environment where trained professionals are available to manage Dennis's complex symptoms.

ANSWERS TO SELF-ASSESSMENT EXERCISE 5.5 (*SEE* P. 55)

1   Is Angelina asking for details regarding diagnosis? How advanced is her dementia? Does she have capacity to understand information and make treatment decisions? Is it important for her to know details in order to give informed consent for appropriate treatment?
2   If treatment is advised and Angelina has capacity to make decisions regarding treatment, she should receive the appropriate information. However, if the information is not essential for treatment decisions and Angelina is not asking, it is acceptable not to initiate discussion about diagnosis if the family believe this would cause distress. Basically, the family must know that if she does ask, it is important that professionals are honest with her.

ANSWER TO SELF-ASSESSMENT EXERCISE 5.6 (*SEE* P. 56)

- It is important to communicate sensitively and in a way which is tailored to the family's understanding. It is necessary for the family to know that their relative is at the end-of-life, the reasons for a decision of this nature at this time and to be reassured that stopping fluids will not impact prognosis. There have been a lot of concerns regarding withdrawing of fluids at the end-of-life relating to the use of the Liverpool Care Pathway (LCP), an issue that has possibly exercised family members more than any other, largely because of the adverse media coverage. In our experience time should be taken to reassure family members that there is no right or wrong position in the debate. The LCP was developed as a care pathway to guide nursing, medical and psychological management in the last days or hours of life. It contains criteria to help identify those people who are dying and guidance about management and relief of symptoms, anticipatory prescribing, and prompts to consider appropriateness of investigations and treatment with medication, fluids or nutrition. Moreover, it prompts communication with the family and consideration of spiritual issues. These are positive procedures, which can be communicated to the concerned family members. While it has provided consistency and *quality* of end-of-life care it has also been used inappropriately in a number of cases, which led to the negative press and its withdrawal from routine care.[13] Consequently, many families have adopted a very critical, almost conspiratorial view of the LCP and similar approaches. This is regrettable, as it was an excellent way of communicating and understanding the complex needs of those who are dying.

CHAPTER 6

End-of-life

Jo Cooper

INTRODUCTION

This chapter discusses end-of-life care in its broadest sense, regardless of diagnosis or place of death. The chapter reviews aspects of a 'good death', place of death and some of the difficulties presented to health professionals and families at the end-of-life.

REFLECTIVE PRACTICE EXERCISE 6.1

Time: 10 minutes
- What do you think constitutes a good death?
- Consider physical, psychological, spiritual, social and family elements.

A good death will mean different things to different people. Such factors as:
➤ choosing the place of death
➤ good pain and symptom management
➤ mending of relationships that may have been difficult or broken
➤ being spiritually at peace with oneself
➤ availability of resources, such as appropriate and timely medications, practical aids to enhance comfort and human resources
➤ effective communication between intra- inter-disciplinary team members.

These are some of the principles representing the features of a good death. Certain factors such as poor pain and symptom management (*see* Chapter 8), lack of choice of place of death, lack of professional teamwork and feelings of a lack of control can lead to a poor or unsuccessful death.[1] As professionals, we may feel that the death of an individual we had cared for had gone particularly well. Pain and distressing symptoms had been managed effectively, the family had been kept well informed by the supporting teams and the individual had died at home – their chosen place of death. However, the family may not feel that this was a good death. It may have been untimely; diagnosis may have been late or mismanaged; poor symptom management and damaged relationships all constitute a suboptimal death. Numerous variables come into play and could cause the family to feel that the death was not as they had planned. A distressing death can also be characterised by the person dying alone, particularly if the family had planned or expected to be present, causing untold anguish for those family members.

REFLECTIVE PRACTICE EXERCISE 6.2

Time: 5 minutes
- Do you feel that 'a good death' is a responsible term for professionals to use?

Masson[2] suggests that the term is inappropriate and idealised, and using the term 'good enough death' may be more achievable and realistic. It is a useful phrase to consider and may be helpful for us to remember when things do not always go to plan. However, we should always aim for the best possible care at the end-of-life, using our knowledge, skills and attitudes in order to prevent unplanned problems.

SELF-ASSESSMENT EXERCISE 6.1

Time: 15 minutes
- Think about the kind of care that you (or someone close to you) would like to have at the end-of-life.
- Make a list of what you feel would be important and meaningful for you.

The National End-of-Life Care Strategy for England[3] defines a good death as:
➤ being treated as an individual with dignity and respect (*see* Chapter 2)
➤ being without pain and other symptoms (*see* Chapter 8)
➤ being in familiar surroundings
➤ being in the company of close family or friends (*see* Chapter 5).

SELF-ASSESSMENT EXERCISE 6.2

Time: 5 minutes
- Does this resonate with you?
- Is there anything you would like to add?

THE CONCEPT OF A GOOD DEATH

The concept of a good death has provoked a great deal of attention in recent months. Governmental (UK) pressures are currently to improve end-of-life care.[4] This leads primarily to the individual having more choice about place of death and to promote a good death, which is paramount not only to the individual themselves and their family, but also for the health professional and teams managing care at the end-of-life.

For many – but not all – individuals, death occurs at the end of a long or chronic ill-health, and is therefore often expected. However, death is still an emotional and physical shock when it happens and the family need ongoing and intensive support at this distressing time. The professional team are present to support and to smooth the way forward for the family who undergo mounting pressures before, during and after the death. It may be more difficult for the family if their relative has not been able to die in their place of choice and this may leave them with an acute sense of guilt, making the bereavement process prolonged and difficult (*see* Chapter 5). In addition, the family will remember this death, and the professional team caring for them, for the rest of their lives, such is the impact at this time. Negative situations may hinder their road to recovery for months or even years.

Since the essence of nursing is to relieve suffering,[5] professionals who continuously witness unrelieved pain or distressing symptoms can feel inadequate, as if they have failed the individual and the family. Professionals involved with caring for those people who are dying may need specialist education, guidance and ongoing support (*see* Chapter 15). We have no way of truly knowing the world of the person who is dying and their family, no way of knowing their past, their experiences, their distress, their losses and sometimes, however much we plan, things do go wrong. For that family, the death may never be a good one.

EARLY ASSESSMENT

Early assessment (*see* Chapter 7), identification and rapid response to symptoms remain paramount when planning for a good death. Pain (and there are many different types, all requiring different approaches and analgesics – *see* Chapter 8) can escalate rapidly, requiring rapid response on the part of the supporting team. People who are dying do not tolerate symptoms easily, due to progressive weakness. This causes undue distress to the person, their family and to the health professional. Continuous review and assessment of pain and symptoms should be regular and ongoing. Situations can change very quickly, in just a few hours, and the team must be prepared for this. Explanations at this time should be given both to the individual and to their family as to why a certain medication is used, what the response might be, and when they can expect palliation. Ensure that the whole intra-/inter-disciplinary team are informed of changes in both condition and medication, so that they are aware of the current situation.

REFLECTIVE PRACTICE EXERCISE 6.3

> **Time: 20 minutes**
> - Does the individual truly have a choice in the type of care and treatment they receive?
> - Does the individual have a choice as to the place in which they would like to die?
> - Reflect on the last person you cared for at the end-of-life (or that you saw being cared for): were they given a choice about place of death, or the type of care they would like to receive. If so, was this achievable for them?

CHOICES

There are times when the wishes and choices of the individual are different to those of their family. Each family member may have a different viewpoint. This is when it is important to bring the family members together to facilitate an empathetic and helpful discussion, in a caring and non-threatening environment. Each person has a story to tell and each person's view is valuable and important. There are occasions when family conflict can arise over aspects of care and/or treatment, and what the family perceive to be the best type of care. This can happen regardless of the place of death.

Case Study 6.1 – Grace – Part I

Grace (72) was dying. She was living in a nursing home, a widow with five adult children. The home staff were happy to keep Grace 'at home', providing they, together with Grace, were supported by the healthcare team. Grace had been comfortable, with minimal pain – managed with a transdermal fentanyl patch. Nausea and vomiting were successfully managed with oral cyclizine. Grace gradually began to lose consciousness – expected by the home staff, but not expected or accepted by some of her family. A syringe driver providing anti-emetics was prescribed, resulting in good management of her symptoms of intractable nausea.

Three members of Grace's family felt that she should have 'a drip' (intravenous fluid), as her mouth was dry, her lips starting to crack and her skin was becoming flaky. Understandably, they felt that she was dehydrated. Grace's two other daughters felt that Grace was comfortable, that she was being well cared for by professionals who knew her and the family well, and that a 'drip' would not help her at this stage of her dying.

Family conflict made it difficult for the home staff to cope, to know what to do, or for them to make a decision alone regarding Grace's care. They contacted the hospice team for help and support.

SELF-ASSESSMENT EXERCISE 6.3

Time: 10 minutes
- As a professional, how would you manage this situation?
- How might you help Grace's family to understand that she was dying and that at this stage, intravenous fluids would be more burdensome than helpful?

Case Study 6.1 – Grace – Part II

A very simple question in this case was all it took to resolve family conflict. The question asked by the health professional was: 'You know your mum better than anyone. What do you think she would have wanted?' Almost immediately, the family agreed that their mum would have wanted to be left in peace – to die in a peaceful and dignified way, with no prolongation of her suffering, with no tubes or drips, unless this would improve her well-being.

Of course, the questions and answers did not just happen! The professional sat, with the family, in Grace's room whilst she slept. They 'chatted' over a cup of tea, getting to know a little about Grace, her life and her loves, from each family member in turn. Each little piece of information built a picture of Grace and reminded the family of past times, and of Grace's character, which sometimes is briefly forgotten or lost in the midst of ongoing distress.

The family, together, understood that a 'drip' would not help Grace. It may even add to her symptoms of nausea and vomiting and the tubes could easily get in the way of getting physically close to Grace. There were other ways the home staff could overcome her dry lips, mouth and flaky skin and the family accepted this, and subsequently became involved with some of these aspects of care. As soon as they realised what 'Mum' would have chosen, their decision was easy, and family unity restored.

Dealing with life, and decisions around death and choice, is not always this simple or easy, but it is a good question to remember to ask. It will not fit all situations. However, in most situations, there is *a* question that guides us … so we can help those involved. The emphasis is on 'listening' and acting on what we hear. The answer is not obvious, it is in the exploration of the problem, uncovering the top layers, and delving underneath. It may involve us taking risks, but unless we do so, we will not help and we will not learn. We cannot 'fix' people's lives, or change them, we can only do our very best to help. Often, as professionals, we enter into complex situations, not knowing what we may find. If we truly listen – and listening is always the key – something happens! We just have to tune in, forget our own concerns and we will find an answer. Often, just by exploring the problem, the person will find his or her own answer. This takes time and skill, but it is a skill that experience brings. The important thing is never to give up.

SELF-ASSESSMENT EXERCISE 6.4

Time: 5 minutes
- How honest are we when people ask us questions about dying?

Most people, but not all, prefer to know, to understand what is happening, so that they are prepared for difficulties that arise during the end-of-life. However, we come back to 'choice'. Not everyone will want candid responses. People have the right to choose how much or how little information they want. If we go too far, they will soon tell us, or show us in their body language. Again, this may cause family conflict. Some families will feel that their relative should not be told the diagnosis, or that they only have 'so long' to live. They feel that the person will not be able to cope. Sometimes this is their own fear and reluctance to deal with the issues that this will bring. During this time, the relatives need just as much support and attention as the individual. Again, it is about exploring, gently and kindly, family perceptions and why they feel as they do; understanding each individual, and taking the time to 'be with'; working alongside the family as the unit of care is an integral part of the essence of caring.

COMMUNICATION STRATEGY

Below are some examples of questions that have been asked by individuals or family members in this author's experience. Guidance is offered as to how the questions could be managed. We all have our own strategies to help, so these are not definitive.

Question 1: How long have I got?

➤ Explore what the person is actually asking you.

➤ Watch their body language, particularly visual expression

➤ Ask: 'How long do you think you may have?' This opens up the question so that you can talk it through and not just give an arbitrary answer.

Question 2: Am I dying?

➤ Ask: 'What makes you ask that question; what's going through your mind?'

➤ Find out what has led up to this – has the person spoken to the doctor recently?

➤ Is it something that has been said, or just thought about?

➤ Ask the person what they think – it gives us time to think, to listen and open up discussion.

Question 3: How will I die?

➤ Some people want to know what to expect. You could ask if they would like to know what to expect.

➤ What are their own expectations? What are they thinking? What are they feeling?

➤ Do they mean what physical symptoms or emotional feelings they might experience, or both of these?

➤ Make sure you have clarified this before talking – explore first.

Question 4: I'm worried about my family. How will they cope?

➤ Find out what the actual and real fear is.

➤ How has the family member coped before when there has been a crisis?

➤ Who will their main support person be?

➤ Be prepared to listen, rather than giving hurried placations.

Question 5: Will I die in pain?

➤ Use exploratory questions.

➤ Tell me about some of your worries about pain.

➤ Is there someone you know who has died in pain?

➤ Is the person talking about physical, emotional or spiritual pain, or all of these?

➤ We can explain about the many and varied types of pharmacological and non-pharmacological methods we use in managing pain.

Question 6: Would you let a dog suffer like this?

➤ Be prepared to sit with this distress and just listen.
➤ Ensure that they feel they have been heard by clarifying some of their thoughts and feelings.
➤ Acknowledge how hard it is for them to watch the person they love die.

REFLECTIVE PRACTICE EXERCISE 6.4

Time: 10 minutes
- For a moment, consider yourself as a spiritual being and consider your own thoughts on the meaning of suffering.

SPIRITUALITY

Spirituality often carries a reference to feelings of 'peace' and dying with 'dignity',[1] with the feelings of being at peace with oneself as a core feature of a good death.[2] Relationships and conflicts from the past can remain distressing for all involved and some form of resolution at the end-of-life is important. This is difficult to achieve but it is implicit, if the individual consents, that we attempt to help. Often, at this time, the individual is more concerned about their family than about themselves, and if they have chosen to receive information regarding their condition, they have time to plan and prepare for their family as well as themselves. We all have our own ideas about dignity (*see* Chapter 2), which can mean different things to different people, and we know when we are being treated with respect. Loss of body image, complex and difficult pain problems, and loss of independence can all be linked to a loss of dignity.[6]

Dignity can be difficult to characterise, but part of caring for each individual means that we must establish how each perceives their own dignity (*see* Chapter 2).

REFLECTIVE PRACTICE EXERCISE 6.5

Time: 30 minutes
Just think how you would like to be treated. For example:
- How would you like to be addressed?
- Would you expect the professional to introduce him- or herself?
- Would you appreciate the professional saying 'thank you for sharing that with me'?
- If you were in a side room, would you appreciate the professional knocking, or asking if it was all right to enter, particularly if family were present?

DYING AT HOME

SELF-ASSESSMENT EXERCISE 6.5

> **Time: 10 minutes**
> - Consider the potential barriers to dying at home.
> - How might these compare with dying in hospital, or nursing and residential care?

Many people choose to die at home. Very few actually do so. 'Home' is the place that the person considers to be his or her home. This may be their own personal home, a nursing or residential home, a family member's home or a hostel where the person has been cared for when experiencing drug- and/or alcohol-related problems (*see* Chapter 14).

One of the problems of end-of-life care at home is the potential lack of resources and rapid responses to symptoms, particularly in rural areas. Insightful community teams will approach the general practitioner/medical doctor and request that drugs needed for end-of-life care are pre-emptively prescribed for the individual, taken to the home and kept in a locked box, ready for use when the time comes. This is especially helpful in terms of 'out of hours' services, when professionals visiting the person may be different from those visiting during normal working hours. Moreover, it can be extremely difficult and frustrating trying to obtain drugs quickly at the weekend when time is of the essence. Symptoms can change rapidly, from hour to hour, and local chemists do not always stock drugs needed for end-of-life care.[1] Keeping drugs at home reassures the individual and the family that they will not be kept waiting in pain or with other symptoms. This also provides the additional benefit of providing peace of mind and reassurance for the visiting professionals. The family should be fully supported at this time and if they 'feel' supported by a trusted team, then dying at home has a much better chance of running smoothly and being successful. If the family want it to work, then it will work. If they are left isolated, feeling unsupported and frightened, then the person is likely to need an admission. However, we need to consider that not all people are going to be cared for at home at the very end, however much they or the family want this. Often people with brain tumours, dementia, difficult chronic illnesses, or where the family is elderly, may prevent a home death. Each situation is different and there is no 'blanket' policy when managing care at the end-of-life.

Wherever a person eventually dies, most time will be spent at home in the last year of life, so providing the best care at home for the final stages will always be important.[7] In addition, the person may have chosen to die at home, but symptoms have become complex and unmanageable and hospital admission is necessary. This can cause an enormous amount of guilt for the family who may have been emotionally planning and preparing for their loved one to die at home. It is important that we listen and acknowledge their feelings of distress and concern, and that they feel heard (*see* Chapter 5).

It is not uncommon for people to change their minds when death approaches or if symptoms become difficult for that person to cope with. Home may become a frightening place to be, and dying at home becomes less important than when they were well.

Case Study 6.2 – Joyce

Joyce (74) was suffering from intractable chest pain, shortness of breath, nausea and agitation. She was cared for at home by her family and recently commenced professional carers. Joyce was told after her hospital admission that she had a chest infection and was given antibiotics, steroids and inhalers, with a transdermal fentanyl patch for pain relief. This was difficult for the family to comprehend as Joyce remained very poorly at home. Joyce had no appetite; she had lost weight, and did not respond to medications for her breathlessness. Her chest and now back pain were well managed using prescribed fentanyl, with OxyNorm for breakthrough pain. Her general practitioner visited when requested and no further hospital admissions were felt necessary. The community nurses provided pressure-relieving aids and Joyce remained physically comfortable with care from her family.

At 0500 one morning, Joyce called for her family. She had struggled out of bed to use the commode, was extremely breathless, pale and feeling agitated and unwell. The family asked her if they could call the paramedics, to which Joyce agreed. Joyce was taken to hospital and admitted under the medical team. The family were told that Joyce was very ill, and would need palliative care, as there was no treatment as such that could be offered 'at this stage'. Although the word 'dying' was not used per se, the family acknowledged and understood that this may be the case. Joyce was diagnosed with a pleural effusion. Her lung was drained and her fentanyl patch increased to compensate for escalating pain.

Joyce had never been able to talk about death or dying. It seemed to frighten her. She had often mentioned in the past that she did not want to die in hospital, but that was as far as her communication went. At this stage, Joyce was happy and content to remain in hospital. She never asked to go home, or protested about where she was. Joyce had always lived in the present moment, was active, and was a loving mother and grandmother.

Because there had been no other diagnosis given, difficult conversations had not taken place with Joyce. Three days before her death she was diagnosed as having lymphoma, with secondary deposits in the lung. For those last three days, Joyce was able to communicate with her family, but still chose not to talk fully or express her feelings around dying. What she did tell her family was that she 'wanted to be with Dad now', so the family knew she had accepted that she was dying. The day prior to her death, she became restless and agitated, with accompanying breathlessness and distress. A syringe driver with analgesia was given, with a sedative to reduce her agitation and feelings of breathlessness. Her symptoms were well managed and Joyce died peacefully in her sleep in the early morning, three days following her diagnosis.

Not knowing her diagnosis until late in her disease did not mean that Joyce did not know that she was dying. She had always been a very strong individual and she died as she had lived, with courage and a strong faith. It was not possible for Joyce to go home to die. Everything happened so quickly, time was very short. Joyce never requested to go home and neither did her family. At the end, Joyce was made physically comfortable and emotionally settled with her family around her for most of the time. Medication was readily available, as was specialist equipment, specialist knowledge and support. The barrier to Joyce dying at home was probably herself. It did not become important to her anymore. What was important for Joyce was that her complex symptoms were well managed; her pain, agitation and breathlessness were all reduced; and those whom she loved and who loved her surrounded her. For Joyce, she understood that she was going to 'a better place'.

RELATIONSHIPS AND COMMUNICATION

Relationships underpin everything that we do … in life generally, personally and professionally. The relationships we form with our colleagues, regardless of what team they represent, the individual for whom we care and the family remain paramount within the practice of caring.

Relationships are built on trust and honesty with each other. They are sometimes fragile and can be broken easily. It takes time, attention and hard work to build good working relationships, but in palliative care it is vital that we take the time and effort to make the relationship work. It has many benefits for all concerned and can help to ensure that we all feel trusted, valued and secure.

SELF-ASSESSMENT EXERCISE 6.6

Time: 10 minutes
- What do you think we need to do to ensure we maintain effective working relationships?

Working with and caring for people who are dying can be distressing and stressful for the health professional. Sitting with a person's distress and feeling their pain can be one of the most difficult aspects of what we do. To make relationships work better, thereby offering a whole team approach providing optimal care to those within our care, we need to:
➤ communicate regularly, openly and effectively with each other. Speak well of our team colleagues and with confidence in their strengths and abilities. If you show the family that you have faith in colleagues, this promotes a good beginning for them
➤ get to know each other as well as possible. Set up regular meetings – these can be brief, but face-to-face meetings are more meaningful than a quick phone call or message. Get to know each other on a human, spiritual level as well as a professional level
➤ acknowledge that we can achieve much more for the person and their family by working cohesively together than we can as individuals

> share our mistakes. We all make them. Talking them through helps others and ourselves to learn. Often our vulnerability is our strength.

Communicating openly with the person who is dying and their family is paramount – each person needs to know what to expect and how we are able to help. Often people tell us that the hospital has said 'there is nothing more we can do'. This causes feelings of rejection and hopelessness. In palliative care, there is always something we can do ... it is a treatment in itself. The goal is *not* to prolong suffering, but to do everything in our knowledge and power that we can to make that person's journey comfortable and well managed. The Gold Standards Framework (GSF) for use in the community has improved communication and teamwork between general practition-ers and health professionals,[8] the primary aim being to improve organisation and increase quality of care for individuals at the end-of-life. The GSF is recommended as a model of good practice. Sometimes we can feel unsure and frightened of open and transparent communication, not just with the person who is dying and their family, but also within the clinical team itself. We may have many concerns that we will not know the answers to the questions we are asked. There is no shame in saying something like 'I don't know the answer to that, but I will take it back to my team and someone will be able to help'. If we do this, it shows that we are acknowledging their difficulty and we are going to do something positive and remedial. Make sure we do go back with the answer – do not keep the person waiting.

Ways of communicating with people who are dying can be learned. Hospices often run study days and workshops and there is always something we can learn. For health professionals who are inexperienced (and we have all been there) we do not always know what we need to know. An experienced colleague can act as a helpful and critical 'friend', reviewing difficult situations and ways of dealing with distress. Clinical supervision is the term used, but this can suggest that only clinical situations need reviewing, and the term 'supervision' can be inappropriate. The relationship we have with a trusted mentor will help us to acknowledge that it is often the dialogue we need to have with people, individuals and family that will smooth the way forward, more than what we actually 'do' in a clinical, hands-on sense. Never be afraid to ask questions yourself. It is the only way we will learn. If you need to ask it, then you can be sure that you will not be the only one wanting to know.

SELF-ASSESSMENT EXERCISE 6.7

Time: 15 minutes

Consider that you are caring for a person at the end-of-life, regardless of their diagnosis.
- What questions are you comfortable with?
- What questions might make you feel uncomfortable or awkward?
- Whom might you approach for help?

Think carefully about your responses.

Acknowledging the culture of the person and their family is important.[7] If you are unsure about this, ask them. People are not offended if they know we need that information in order to help them. People are more likely to feel offended if we *do not* ask. People all differ in their needs regarding family involvement; some will accept help from the family, others may not. It is important that we show respect, sensitivity and acknowledge the person's choice. Cultural issues may create barriers to good communication, which can lead to feelings of discrimination and lack of empathy (*see* Chapter 4).[9] Everyone will have their own traditional values, and we must have respect and understanding when caring for people from different cultures.

When we talk about 'the family', this can mean different things to different people. It does not necessarily mean blood relatives. It could be same sex partners, close friends or a neighbour but they may be considered to be that person's family. It is always prudent to check just how much information the family want. Some families will want to know everything, others virtually nothing. Take a systematic approach, just a little at a time, and gauge the reactions. Again, never be afraid to ask. Most will choose to have information, given in lay terms, so that they know what to expect. Our presence within the home is valuable, in terms of supportive and empathic care, whatever position in the team we are. We may not always be needed to perform 'a task', but being ourselves and being alongside the family is of paramount importance when giving end-of-life care.

There is often a long and unpredictable journey for people experiencing mental health problems. Providing care at the end-of-life for people experiencing dementia and other mental health problems can present a raft of challenging situations, involving the individual, the family and the professionals (*see* Chapters 9, 10, 11 and 12). Communication can be stressful and constrained for the individual, who may forget facts or be unable to express them. People experiencing dementia can encounter problems comparable with those of people who have a cancer diagnosis, but the former experience a lower quality of care at the end-of-life.[10,11] The ability to make an informed choice and decisions about type and place of care may be denied. The family need to be involved at every point in their journey and looked upon as experts in that person's care. Ongoing assessment and review of symptoms is just as important as with any ill-health, and changes managed appropriately and responsibly. A slow decline in physical function and ability enables general practitioners/medical doctors to recognise the nearness of end-of-life.[12] The family often express fears about the person's diminishing food intake, how the person will die and how they will recognise that the end-of-life is approaching. These issues will need exploration with the family and time and advice should be given to help them to understand what it is they will be facing. The needs of the family are sometimes overlooked and a conscious effort to talk – and to listen – regularly is needed wherever end-of-life care is taking place. If admission to hospital is needed, the family should be invited to help with care, if they choose and are willing to do so.

END-OF-LIFE

SELF-ASSESSMENT EXERCISE 6.8

Time: 5 minutes
- Can you identify some of the common features indicating that the end-of-life is approaching?

It is often difficult to know just when the end-of-life is near. Some people will exhibit the classic signs others may not. The following is a guide and is considered normal progression. However, this can be a frightening time for the family if they have not been well prepared:

➤ loss of appetite
➤ reduction in oral intake
➤ loss of interest in their surroundings and social withdrawal
➤ continuing weight loss
➤ wanting to remain in bed
➤ decline in the ability to communicate.

Some people at the end-of-life will be too ill to make decisions about their care. However, Jeffries[6] reminds us that the end-of-life offers a last opportunity to make choices. It is important to remember that even if communication is difficult, we must try to obtain the individual's agreement for care required. As the person becomes less attentive, the family will become more involved, acting on that person's behalf.

CONCLUSION

Good end-of-life care should be available in all settings, regardless of diagnosis. The individual and the family remain the central focus of care with therapeutic relationships and effective communication as the foundation for providing this care. We need knowledge, skills, the right attitude, and attention to the smallest detail to make someone's care at the end-of-life a 'good' experience. Families need and deserve help with preparation in knowing what to expect when a person dies, both emotionally and physically. An important point for us to consider is that each individual should feel heard, their views valued, so taking time to listen and act on what we hear, plays an important role for each person and family member. We need to be able to respond quickly to physical and emotional symptoms, with understanding, kindness and compassion (*see* Chapter 2).

We must, in doing this work, also take care of each other and ourselves. This is not being narrow; it has far-reaching and positive effects for those within our care. Treat ourselves with compassion – know our colleagues and ourselves – learn about who we are, for working with people, human being to human being, teaches us much about ourselves. We can consciously use this learning to help others, giving the best possible care to those individuals who are entering the final stage in the journey of life.

REFERENCES

1 Griggs C. Community nurses' perception of a good death: a qualitative exploratory study. *International Journal of Palliative Nursing.* 2010; **16**: 139–48.

2 Masson JD. Non-professional perceptions of 'good death': a study of the views of hospice care patients and relatives of deceased hospice care patients. *Mortality.* 2002; 7: 191–209.

3 Department of Health. *End of Life Care Strategy: promoting high quality care for all adults at the end of life.* London: Department of Health; 2008. Available at: www.gov.uk/government/publica tions/end-of-life-care-strategy-promoting-high-quality-care-for-adults-at-the-end-of-their-life (accessed 13 February 2014).

4 The National Council for Palliative Care. *End of Life Care Strategy.* London: The National Council for Palliative Care; 2006. Available at: www.ncpc.org.uk/sites/default/files/NCPC_EoLC_ Submission.pdf (accessed 13 February 2014).

5 Beauchamp TL, Childress JF. *Principles of Biomedical Ethics.* 5th ed. New York: Oxford University Press; 2001.

6 Jeffrey D. *Patient-centred Ethics and Communication at the End of Life.* Oxford: Radcliffe Publishing; 2006. pp. 24, 28.

7 Social Care Institute for Excellence, Rutter D, Holmes P. *Dying Well at Home: the case for inte-grated working.* London: Social Care Institute for Excellence; 2013. Available at: www.scie.org. uk/publications/guides/guide48/files/guide48.pdf (accessed 13 February 2014.

8 Mahmood-Yousuf K, Munday D, King N, *et al.* Interprofessional relationships and communi-cation in primary palliative care: impact of the Gold Standard Framework. *British Journal of General Practice.* 2008; **58**: 256–63.

9 Eshiett Mu-A, Parry EHO. Migrants and health: a cultural dilemma. *Clinical Medicine.* 2003; **3**: 229–31.

10 Mitchell S, Kiely D, Hamel MB. Dying with advanced dementia in the nursing home. *Archives of Internal Medicine.* 2004; **164**: 321–6.

11 Sampson EL, Gould V, Lee D, *et al.* Differences in care received by patients with and without dementia who died during acute hospital admission: a retrospective case note study. *Age and Ageing.* 2006; **35**: 187–9.

12 Grisaffi K, Robinson L. Timing of end of life care in dementia: difficulties and dilemmas for GPs. *Journal of Dementia Care.* 2010; **18**: 36–9.

TO LEARN MORE

- Cooper DB and Cooper J. *Palliative Care within Mental Health: principles and philosophy.* London: Radcliffe Publishing; 2012.

- Cooper J. *Stepping in to Palliative Care: care and practice.* 2nd ed. Oxford: Radcliffe Publishing; 2006.

- Cooper J. *Stepping in to Palliative Care: relationships and responses.* 2nd ed. Oxford: Radcliffe Publishing; 2006.

- Jeffries D. *Patient-centred Ethics and Communication at the End of Life.* Oxford: Radcliffe Publishing; 2006.

- Rinpoche S. *The Tibetan Book of Living and Dying: a spiritual classic from one of the foremost interpreters of Tibetan Buddhism to the West.* Edited by Gaffney P, Harvey A. London/Sydney/ Auckland/Johannesburg: Rider: 2008.

CHAPTER 7

Assessment

John R Ashcroft

INTRODUCTION

The World Health Organization defines palliative care as:

> an approach which improves the quality of life of patients and their families facing life-threatening illness, through the prevention, assessment and treatment of pain and other physical, psychosocial and spiritual problems.[1]

REFLECTIVE PRACTICE EXERCISE 7.1

Time: 10 minutes

Consider your own practice area:

- How frequently do you provide palliative care to individuals experiencing serious and enduring mental health problems?
- Think carefully – has this been a conscious or unconscious act?

The concept of palliative care has evolved and it is becoming increasingly apparent that the approach used in palliative care need not necessarily be for people approaching the end of their life.

KEY POINT 7.1

The term 'palliative care' is the alleviation of suffering regardless of the availability of cure or the stage of ill-health.

It is intended that through the relief of symptoms the individual and their family can achieve the best quality of life possible.

SELF-ASSESSMENT EXERCISE 7.1

Time: 5 minutes
What would you consider to be the key principles in mental health care?

Mental health nursing students frequently argue that they engage in the key principles of palliative care[2] and the similarity in philosophy between palliative care and mental health practice has been described and includes:[3]

➤ person-centred practice
➤ relationship-based connectedness
➤ a belief in compassionate, holistic care
➤ respect for autonomy and choice
➤ quality of life issues
➤ family as the unit of care
➤ the need for a democratic and intra-/inter-discipline work team.

SELF-ASSESSMENT EXERCISE 7.2

Time: 10 minutes
- What skills, including interpersonal skills, are needed to 'find out' (assess) all about an individual so you can really help them?
- Think about 'who' the person is, not what diagnosis he or she may have.

ASSESSMENT IN SERIOUS AND ENDURING MENTAL HEALTH

Assessment has been described as the cornerstone of effective mental health practice[4] and there is evidence to suggest that the assessment process itself can be therapeutic.[5]

REFLECTIVE PRACTICE EXERCISE 7.2

Time: 10 minutes
- Reflect on the above statement.
- Write down how you think the assessment process can be therapeutic to:
  - the individual
  - you as the assessor.

Upon presentation to mental health services, assessment is often focused on determining current symptoms in order to make a 'diagnosis'. An individual may be seen by a number of professionals and be asked about the history and duration of their symptoms, in addition to receiving mental and physical examination.

SELF-ASSESSMENT EXERCISE 7.3

> **Time: 5 minutes**
> Whilst acknowledging the above is useful and necessary information for the professional, how helpful is it to the individual who may be distressed, frightened, angry, withdrawn?

Psychotropic medication may be prescribed and/or psychosocial intervention arranged. The success or failure of treatment is often determined by the reduction or continued presence of the initial presenting symptoms. Laing[6] termed this approach the *medical model*, an approach to disease that aims to find medical treatments for diagnosed symptoms *in the presence of evident pathology*.

In most medical specialties, physical examination and investigation will typically precede diagnosis. With the exception of physical trauma and infectious diseases, the exact cause of disease is often unknown, unclear, or believed to be multi-factorial. However, even if the cause of disease is unclear, pathology, in terms of the physical manifestations of the cause, is usually evident before a diagnosis is made and treatment initiated. Examples include hypertension, many cancers, and neurological disorders. Treatment is then often focused upon symptom relief *in addition* to attempts made to reverse physiological change (e.g. inflammation).

DIAGNOSIS IN SERIOUS AND ENDURING MENTAL HEALTH

Medical diagnosis and treatment in mental health is fundamentally different to other specialties. Diagnosis is made based on collections of symptoms (syndromes) occurring together in a predictable manner and treatment is focused on alleviating these symptoms as opposed to tackling pathology. In this way, there is an assumption that there are underlying cause(s) for the syndromes, yet to be discovered. It was the German psychiatrist Emil Kraeplin who first coined this idea and on whose work current psychiatry classification systems (ICD-10[7] and DSM-1V[8]) are still based.[9]

SELF-ASSESSMENT EXERCISE 7.4

> **Time: 5 minutes**
> If we use a classification system to uncover problems, how can this help us to get to 'know' the 'person'?

ICD-10 and DSM-1V both acknowledge the limitations of the current classification systems and describe how professionals should consider that individuals sharing a diagnosis are likely to be heterogeneous even in regard to the defining features of the diagnosis.[7,8]

A common misconception is that the classification of mental disorders classifies people, when actually it is the disorders that are being classified. It is the individual who experiences the symptoms of schizophrenia (schizophrenia being a cluster of many possible symptoms that are regularly seen together) and all that this entails, as opposed to the person being 'a schizophrenic'.

It has been argued that given the absence of evident pathology in mental ill-health (with the exception of a number of neuropsychiatric disorders) and that treatment essentially involves the alleviation of subjectively distressing mental states, the application of a medical model or approach to such treatment symptoms is inappropriate.[6]

Many professionals are perturbed by the suggestion that psychiatric diagnosis is not diagnosis in the true sense of the word, believing that this suggests that mental 'ill' health, as a concept, does not exist. However, it should be noted that the absence of the clinical and physical manifestations of disease is not synonymous with the absence of ill-health.

Health has been defined as:

> a state of complete physical, mental, and social well-being and not simply
> the absence of disease or infirmity.[10]

The presence of mental health symptoms, therefore, are sufficient evidence of 'ill' health.

SUBJECTIVE EXPERIENCE

> **KEY POINT 7.2**
>
> Remember that what the assessing professional deems as important may not be so to the individual presenting with symptoms.

The assessor may be attempting to illicit psychopathology (i.e. abnormal experiences, cognition and behaviour) in an attempt to make a diagnosis, whereas the person experiencing symptoms wishes to convey their subjective experience and distress. The objective description or label may be the same, yet the subjective experience completely different. The philosophical concept of *qualia* refers to the subjectivity of perceptual experiences and the near impossibility to relay that experience verbally to others.[11] Although we label colours as red, green or blue, for example, how can I be confident that my blue is your blue?

In this context reality is determined through an individual's thoughts and their subjective perceptual experiences as opposed to objective observation. The same may be applied to subjective emotional experiences. Any two individuals with identical objectively described mental health symptoms, and indeed identical expression of these symptoms, may have completely different subjective experiences.

KEY POINT 7.3

The approach to each person needs to be tailored towards his or her individual needs rather than simply aimed at alleviating the symptoms as listed in any categorical diagnostic classification system.

THE PALLIATIVE CARE APPROACH TO SERIOUS AND ENDURING MENTAL HEALTH

KEY POINT 7.4

Although palliative care is typically reserved for individuals with terminal ill-health, it could be argued that given the treatment of most medical disorders involves the alleviation of symptoms as opposed to cure, all disease could be treated using a palliative approach.

However, financial and time constraints often mean that treatment is focused upon alleviation of presenting symptoms even though physical ill-health is likely to have impacted on other aspects of the individual's life, particularly if ill-health has been chronic. Similarly, it is appreciated that mental health symptoms do not take place in isolation and an eclectic, holistic, person-centred approach to assessment is essential. An understanding and appreciation of this connection is paramount if measures are to be put in place to improve quality of life of an individual experiencing serious and enduring mental health symptoms.

SELF-ASSESSMENT EXERCISE 7.5

Time: 5 minutes
How would you assess what the quality of life is for the person, and what this means for him or her?

An individual experiencing serious and enduring mental health concerns and dilemmas may remain in contact with mental health services for years if not decades. Throughout this period the person may receive a number of diagnostic labels and it may be assumed (falsely) that the original diagnosis was inaccurate. However, if the limitations of the current diagnostic classification system are recognised (i.e. that the diagnosis of psychiatric disorders is a *descriptive* process and makes no reference to the cause of illness) it is to be *expected* that diagnosis will change over time in accordance with the individual's needs and variable presenting symptoms.

A diagnosis based on *cause* would be less likely to change over time. As cause of mental ill-health is usually unknown, this is used as a rationale for employing alternative models and treatment approaches to mental health symptoms. Medical diagnosis and assessment often describes an individual's presentation *at one point in time*, i.e. in cross-section. Although possibly helpful in relaying information to other professionals, a particular diagnostic label is at best incomplete and may possibly, at worst, be stigmatising. Thus additional information is required to gain an understanding of the unique problems of the individual experiencing serious and enduring mental health symptoms.

A longitudinal assessment is preferable to determine the impact of symptoms on various facets of a person's life over often significant periods of time. Therefore the person-centred approach recognises that regardless of diagnosis an individual will have different needs at different phases of her or his ill-health.

KEY POINT 7.5

Families and carers require considerable support throughout and will have variable needs themselves.

Assessment therefore needs to reflect this and is a continuous and ongoing dynamic process.

ASSESSMENT

What is the aim of assessment?

Ultimately the purpose of assessment is to find out what needs to be done to improve an individual's quality of life and to determine how this is best done in relation to the unique circumstances of the individual being assessed.

The assessing professional aims to:
➤ gather information about the:
  — person
  — family
  — illness
  — associated problems[12]
➤ identify factors associated with the health problems[12]
➤ highlight a person's coping strategies and to explore their strengths and weaknesses.[12]

REFLECTIVE PRACTICE EXERCISE 7.3

Time: 15 minutes
Think about how you find out the above information.
● Do you assess a person using a questionnaire, filling in or ticking appropriate boxes?
● Do you ask the person a series of questions, making notes about what you feel is important?
● Do you ask a few leading questions, and then listen carefully to the person's story?

- If you write down any assessment details, and if so, do you give a copy to the person?
- Do you do something else?
- Which method do you feel would help you and the individual the most – and why? Think long-term.

When should assessment occur?

Key recommendation 2 of NICE guidelines states that:

> assessment and discussion of patients' needs for physical, psychological, social, spiritual and financial support should be undertaken at key points (such as at diagnosis; at commencement, during and at the end of treatment; at relapse; and when death is approaching).[13]

Where should assessment take place?

The assessment may be lengthy, dependent upon the complexity of issues discussed and the person's ability (or desire) to relay information. Therefore measures should be taken to ensure that assessment takes place in a private yet safe and comfortable environment. Assessment does not have to be completed all at once. Tailor the length of the assessment to the individual's needs. Assessment is an ongoing procedure and not a 'one-off' exercise.

SELF-ASSESSMENT EXERCISE 7.6

Time: 5 minutes

How could the environment be manipulated in order to make it therapeutic (therapeutic environment)?

Distractions and unnecessary interruptions should be avoided. The assessing professional should book sufficient time in their diary for assessment to take place. Too much allocated time is preferable to not enough.

KEY POINT 7.6

Clock-watching does not encourage an individual to engage with the assessment process. To gain trust an individual needs to feel that they are listened to, and their story is important.

A rushed assessment when an individual is made to feel that another issue is pending is unlikely to be productive.

Who should perform the assessment?

It is of paramount importance that the assessor is a professional with an appropriate level of knowledge of serious and enduring mental health problems, the many manifestations, and the various potential impacts. The assessor needs to be competent in key aspects of the assessment process and have developed the skills needed.

REFLECTIVE PRACTICE EXERCISE 7.4

Time: 5 minutes
- How could you develop and improve your own skills of assessment?
- What changes do you need to make?

This has huge implications in terms of an individual's first contact with services and triage. A lack of expertise and experience in the assessor at this point could lead to people experiencing mental health problems not being recognised as needing assistance.

SELF-ASSESSMENT EXERCISE 7.7

Time: 5 minutes
What should assessment include?

Each person has their own story, which we should encourage them to tell – in their own words and their own time, giving them time and space in which to tell. You will then know what information and cues are important to act on and how you will act.

What assessment skills should be developed?

Empathy

The concept of empathy is a clinical instrument that needs to be used with skill to measure another person's internal subjective state using the observer's own capacity for emotional and cognitive experience as a yardstick.[14] Empathy should be distinguished from sympathy, which implies that the observer *feels sorry for* the observed. Of course the two are not mutually exclusive, although sympathy may impact on the assessor's ability to empathise.

The assessor's ability to understand a person's experience from the person's point of view – *empathy* – is preferable as an assessment skill than to imagine how the assessor would feel in the same situation – *sympathy*.

> You never really understand a person until you consider things from his point of view … until you climb into his skin and walk around in it.[15]

An understanding of non-verbal communication

Non-verbal communication can be used to infer the subjective emotional state and thought processes of an individual. Examples include:

➤ **facial expressions** – e.g. smiling, frowning
➤ **gestures** – e.g. waving, pointing
➤ **paralinguistics** – refers to vocal communication that is separate from language, e.g. tone, volume, inflection, pitch
➤ **body language (gestures, posture, eye gaze)** – e.g.:
  — avoidance of eye contact or an excessive held gaze may be significant
  — pointing may be evidence of aggression
  — a slumped, withdrawn posture may signify low mood
➤ **proxemics** – refers to personal space and is often dependent on culture, gender and social situation[16]
➤ **haptics** – refers to communication through touch. When used in a socially appropriate situation touch may be used to communicate affection, sympathy or fear, for example, although when used in the wrong context it may suggest over-familiarity
➤ **appearance** – our dress sense, hairstyle, hair colour, cleanliness, presence of tattoos may all be considered a means of non-verbal communication, particularly if there is a radical change in behaviour over a period. The ongoing continuous nature of assessment will enable such changes to be noticed.

We all make use of verbal and non-verbal communication in our personal lives, often on an unconscious level. The assessor should be aware, however, that non-verbal communication and gestures can vary considerably between cultures (*see* Chapter 4 and below on cultural consideration). In addition, it should be noted that mental ill-health and its treatment can have a huge impact upon non-verbal communication *within* a given culture. For example, individuals experiencing side effects of Parkinsonism secondary to the use of antipsychotic medication often have a paucity of facial expression and spontaneous movement. Moreover, individuals diagnosed with dementia, or who have suffered traumatic brain injury, may have paralinguistic changes with alteration in prosody (intonation).

Communication is a two-way process

The professional who is *aware* of his or her non-verbal conversational ability has a potentially extremely effective tool for use in the establishment of rapport, trust and the therapeutic relationship.[12] Thus it may be beneficial in this regard to:

➤ maintain a relaxed body posture
➤ use appropriate eye contact
➤ maintain physical 'openness'
➤ use appropriate relaxed facial expressions
➤ nod head in encouragement.[12]

Appropriate use of silences
➤ Allows time for the assessing professional and individual to collect their thoughts.
➤ May encourage those less communicative individuals to 'open up' and provide information.[12]

Sometimes, silence can feel uncomfortable. We often feel we need to speak, rather than allow that silence. Silence gives individuals and professionals time to gather their thoughts and think about how to express what they feel.

Active listening
➤ Assists in creating a therapeutic relationship.
➤ Enables the individual to begin to share their world.
➤ Allows an individual sufficient time to talk and complete statements before asking further questions or making comments.[12]

How long should assessment take?

KEY POINT 7.7
As long as it takes.

The ongoing nature of assessment allows for information to be gathered over more than one session.

KEY POINT 7.8
A balance needs to be found between gathering too much information at one time with the risk of overloading an individual and allowing insufficient time for a person to relay their story, including their fears and expectations.

What should assessment include?

Case Study 7.1 – Mike – Part I

Mike, 22, has experienced significant anxiety when in social situations since his early teenage years. He has gradually become more socially withdrawn and isolated. His alcohol use has increased over recent months and he smokes 20 cigarettes a day, although this may double when he drinks. He is presently unemployed and lives alone. Mike achieved good grades at school at GCSE and A levels although dropped out of university after two months. Mike was studying psychology and was regularly required to give presentations in tutorials and seminars. His anxiety significantly increased, with consequent avoidance of situations where he was expected to speak publicly. He felt unable to discuss his situation with tutors and decided not to return after the first semester break. Mike's mood became increasingly low. After attending his general practitioner (GP) for a chest infection, Mike also mentioned his symptoms of low mood, anxiety and disturbed sleep. Selective serotonin re-uptake inhibitors (SSRIs) – a class of antidepressant drugs initially used to treat symptoms of depression although which are now widely used to treat a variety of conditions including anxiety, panic, obsessive compulsive and personality disorders – were commenced and a referral made to mental health services after Mike reported experiencing increasingly frequent thoughts of suicide. After taking medication for several days, he discontinued treatment and failed to attend the appointment offered due to significant anticipatory anxiety.

SELF-ASSESSMENT EXERCISE 7.8

Time: 5 minutes
What do you need to know about Mike and his family relationships in order to really help and work alongside him?

Case Study 7.1 – Mike – Part II
Primary issues
- Descriptive terms to define Mike's symptoms such as depression or social phobia do not sufficiently relay the debilitating impact that these symptoms have had on his life.
- Mike feels that his main concerns at present are no longer his symptoms of anxiety and low mood per se but rather the impact that they have had on his personal life.

An assessment of physical health
Mike's alcohol and cigarette use had significantly increased over several months. A recent chest infection was believed to be related to an increase in smoking.

There is much evidence to suggest that those experiencing serious and enduring mental health problems have significantly increased morbidity and an increased mortality risk.[17,18] For example, there is evidence that depression may be an independent risk factor for heart disease in men,[19] an association independent of smoking status, diabetes, hypertension and deprivation score.[19] In addition, there is a significantly increased risk of drug and alcohol use in individuals experiencing serious and enduring mental health,[20] along with the physical health complications associated with their use.

Assessment of social and interpersonal relationships
Mike has become increasingly socially isolated and he has lost contact from friends he made at school. His unwillingness to attend social events has led to him no longer

being invited. Although SSRI medication may well be of benefit in terms of mild alleviation of current symptoms, there needs to be an appreciation of the longer term impact of Mike's symptoms on his life. His only regular social contacts are those members of his immediate family, although Mike also avoids family gatherings.

Although it is the individual experiencing serious and enduring mental health problems who personally experiences the symptoms, the impact of the experience will extend to the individual's family, friends and other members of their support network.

An assessment of the individual's financial situation

In Mike's particular case his symptoms have significantly affected his ability to gain employment due to his avoidance of anxiety-provoking interviews.

An assessment of the importance of religion or spirituality to the individual

A person may turn away from their religious beliefs or have difficulty incorporating their experience into pre-existing belief systems. The individual may ask 'why me?' Alternatively, a person may find solace through their faith or particular belief.

An assessment of the impact of mental health symptoms on the individual's sexuality

Medication side effects are associated with decreased libido, ejaculation difficulty and erection difficulties in men.[21] Men in particular are often reluctant to reveal or discuss such issues, with potentially devastating consequences.

The symptoms may strain relationships and possibly lead to relationship breakdown. Confidence and self-esteem may be affected. The person may discontinue medication with a consequent deterioration in mental health. Moreover, the individual may seek to self-medicate with illicit substances or potentially harmful black-market sexual performance-enhancing drugs.

An assessment of the impact of serious and enduring mental ill-health on psychological well-being

Serious and enduring mental ill-health itself is a risk factor for further mental health symptoms and there is evidence to suggest that the prevalence of psychiatric comorbidity is extremely high.[22] Mike's low mood appears to have developed secondary to his symptoms of anxiety.

Although an individual may have been diagnosed with a particular mental disorder, this does not render her or him immune to the development of further psychological disturbance, which of course may itself exacerbate pre-existing symptoms.

The risk of suicide in those experiencing schizophrenia symptoms is significantly higher than the general population,[23] believed to be related to the development of depression secondary to psychotic symptoms and associated with the use of illicit substances and/or alcohol.

KEY POINT 7.9

- *All* aspects of an individual's life are closely related.
- A problem in one area is likely to lead to difficulties in another, as issues do not occur in isolation. The physical, mental and social aspects of life are often closely interconnected.
- This increases the risk that an individual experiencing serious and enduring mental health may at some point decide to attempt to take his or her own life.

Case Study 7.1 – Mike – Part III

Mike became increasingly isolated and detached himself from family members and friends, who began to visit less regularly. His alcohol use continued to increase and his physical health began to suffer. On one occasion, while intoxicated, he visited the local off-licence to purchase more alcohol and got into an altercation with a member of the public. The shop owner, fearful that the situation, now taking place outside of the shop, was getting out of hand, called the police. Mike had been becoming increasingly self-conscious and paranoid whilst out in public, although he rarely ventured outdoors other than for self-determined essentials.

The police arrested Mike, and due to his suspicious presentation, deemed that he required psychiatric assessment. He was taken to a place of safety and assessed by a psychiatrist, who found Mike to be suspicious and hostile. Mike felt he had not been treated fairly, and simply wished to return home.

SELF-ASSESSMENT EXERCISE 7.9

Time: 5 minutes
What do you feel could be contributing to Mike's feelings of paranoia?

Case Study 7.1 – Mike – Part IV

Mike expressed a belief that he was being victimised and that there was a conspiracy against him involving the police and the assessing psychiatrist. His aggressive behaviour continued. When sober, a Mental Health Act assessment was arranged and the professionals agreed that he may be experiencing a psychotic illness. Mike was detained under Section 2 of the UK Mental Health Act 1983 – a 28-day assessment order.[24]

Mike agreed to take medication on the ward, his symptoms of paranoia and anxiety appeared to resolve, and the section was rescinded. Mike was discharged with appropriate aftercare. A tentative diagnosis of schizophrenia was made. However, Mike did not feel he needed the medication and disputed the diagnosis of schizophrenia.

SELF-ASSESSMENT EXERCISE 7.10

Time: 5 minutes

What factors, other than medication, may have contributed to the resolution of Mike's symptoms?

Case Study 7.1 – Mike – Part V

Despite continuing to the take medication in the community, Mike relapsed on two occasions following discharge, each occasion resulting in a hospital admission. Relapses consisted of excessive alcohol consumption associated with suspicious and aggressive behaviour. On one occasion Mike expressed suicidal ideation.

SELF-ASSESSMENT EXERCISE 7.11

Time: 4 minutes

What could be the cause for Mike's relapse?

Case Study 7.1 – Mike – Part VI

Mike was again discharged to the community and significant efforts are being made for him to engage in community activities through attendance at local community groups. Following referral Mike has been attending cognitive behavioural therapy sessions focused on anxiety management and confidence building and he has found this helpful. Mike now feels that at some point he would like to return to college.

CULTURAL CONSIDERATIONS (*SEE* CHAPTER 4)

We live in a diverse, multicultural and multi-faith society. The subject of transcultural health is huge, and significant literature has been written both on the subject as a whole and on issues more specifically relating to mental health. An excellent example and the most used at an international level is the Purnell Model (*see* Chapter 4). There may be considerable variation in the presentation of individuals with physical or mental health problems from different cultural backgrounds

Although there is minimal evidence to suggest that the experience of pain varies across cultures, studies have found that the *expression* of pain does.[25,26] This may also extend to the expression of distress in general (*mental pain*). For example, in certain cultures depressive ill-health may manifest as somatic symptoms, such as headache, general malaise or abdominal discomfort, rather than subjective sadness or emotional disturbance.[27]

In addition to the variable cultural *expression* or manifestation of symptoms is the cultural *explanation* of symptoms, which may in some instances appear to be delusional. The assessing professional needs to be aware that a belief system deemed to be abnormal in one culture may be acceptable in another. A belief in magic, spirits or demonic possession may be a culturally acceptable explanation for serious anxiety, panic attacks and obsessive-compulsive symptoms in some societies.

Historically there has been a tendency in the UK to make a diagnosis of schizophrenia more readily in particular cultural groups such as Afro-Carribeans.[28] Rather than representing a difference in the incidence of schizophrenia, this is likely to reflect a lack of appreciation of cultural differences. Moreover, gestures in one culture may have a completely different meaning in another. For example, in England tapping the side of the nose with index finger is a signal for secrecy although in Italy it is understood as a friendly warning to take care.[29]

Subculture and cultural change

Indeed, *within societies* what is deemed to be acceptable in terms of behaviour, belief and mode of communication may change over time. Culture, inclusive of verbal and non-verbal communication, is not static. In the US, homosexuality was considered to be a mental disorder until its removal as a classified mental disorder was agreed in 1973.[30] An older generation may deem the behaviour of a younger generation to be inherently rude, disruptive or possibly immoral.

The acceptability of alcohol and substance use can be influenced by culture. For example, the use of hallucinogens is recognised as part of religious rituals in some societies[31] and the use of substances within the dance music scene is so prevalent as to possibly constitute a subculture.[32]

It may be extremely challenging for the assessing professional to evaluate an individual from a different ethnicity. The issue may be compounded if there is a language barrier, for example if the individual is a recent immigrant or asylum seeker.

Although possibly helpful to some, a list of dos and don'ts may be overwhelming for the assessing professional, possibly leading to avoidance of key issues in some instances. But for those who would find a list helpful as an educational tool, *see* Box 7.1, pp. 94–8. However, assessment tools are merely memory aids that are helpful in certain situations, thus it needs to be remembered when using assessment tools that these are aids and do not replace person-centred assessment and clinical knowledge in one-to-one contact.

The assessing professional cannot be expected to know every nuance and aspect of each culture and religious denomination likely to be encountered. However, several suggestions and recommendations may be helpful to avoid perceived misconceptions and differences in beliefs and values.

➤ Be aware of stereotyping and avoid making assumptions.
  — If cultural differences between assessor and individual with mental health symptoms are not taken into account, the assessment is prone to potentially significant errors.[33]

➤ If in doubt, ASK.
  — It is perfectly acceptable to ask how a person wishes to be addressed or whether he or she is comfortable discussing a particular topic.
➤ Use interpreters when necessary.
  — Where language difficulties are apparent, the use of interpreters is advantageous. Where possible, the interpreter should share a cultural background with the individual being assessed rather than simply speaking their language.
  — The assessing professional should be aware of the potential pitfalls and errors in the use of interpreters.[34] Information and context may be lost in translation through the addition, alteration, substitution or omission of detail, for example.
  — The use of family members as interpreters should be avoided and ideally reserved for emergencies only. The reasons are all the same as the potential pitfalls and errors as stated below. However, they are more likely to occur voluntarily for three possible reasons:
    1 the individual may be less willing to relay sensitive information to a family member than an interpreter
    2 the interpreting family member may be unwilling to relay perceived sensitive family details and information to the assessing professional
    3 the use of minors as interpreters is unethical due to the potentially rather sensitive nature of the subject matter likely to be discussed, which may be upsetting or disturbing for younger children, teenagers or young adults.

These factors in extreme circumstances could possibly render the interpretation meaningless if important information has in effect been voluntarily censored.

In addition to recognisable mental health symptoms manifesting in individuals from different cultures in different ways, a number of *culture-bound syndromes* have been described.[35,36] This term refers to mental health issues that may occur only in specific cultures. Much has been written on the subject and many such syndromes have been described.[36] Examples include:

➤ **amok** – from the Malay meaning 'to engage furiously in battle'. Seen in South East Asia and associated with outbursts of aggressive and extremely violent behaviour following a period of depression or anxiety
➤ **koro** – seen in males of South East Asia and associated with a fear or delusion that the penis has retracted into the abdomen or shrunk and that death is shortly to occur
➤ **anorexia nervosa** – has been regarded by some as a culture-bound syndrome, given that it is almost exclusively seen in Western cultures or in those cultures heavily influenced by them.[37]

The topic is highly controversial, however, and some argue that the mental health issues represent local variations of recognised Western disorders as defined by ICD-10[7] and DSM-IV[8] classification systems, whereas others believe that they represent discrete culture-specific entities. Nevertheless, modern society consists of extremely diverse immigrant groups and the assessing professional may be faced with an individual displaying behaviour uncharacteristic of the indigenous culture. The benefits of an increased awareness of the concept of culture-bound syndromes are therefore clear for professionals serving an increasingly diverse population.

CONCLUSION AND PRIMARY ISSUES

➤ The term 'palliative care' is frequently being used more and more to refer to the alleviation of suffering regardless of the availability of cure or the stage of ill-health.

➤ The physical, mental and social aspects of life are often closely interconnected.

➤ A problem in one area is likely to lead to difficulties in another, as issues do not occur in isolation.

➤ Ultimately the purpose of assessment is to find out what needs to be done to improve an individual's quality of life and to determine how this is best done in relation to the unique circumstances of the individual being assessed.

➤ The professional who is aware of his or her non-verbal communicational ability has a potentially extremely effective tool for use in the establishment of rapport, trust and the therapeutic relationship.

➤ We live in a diverse, multicultural and multi-faith society. There may be considerable variation in the presentation of individuals with physical or mental health problems from different cultural backgrounds.

REFERENCES

1 World Health Organization. *WHO Definition of Palliative Care*. Geneva: World Health Organization; 1990.

2 Black C, Hanson E, Cutcliffe J, *et al*. Palliative care nurses and mental health nurses: sharing common ground? *International Journal of Palliative Nursing*. 2001; **7**: 17–23.

3 McGrath P, Holewa H. Mental health and palliative care: exploring the ideological interface. *International Journal of Psychosocial Rehabilitation*. 2004; **9**: 107–19.

4 Gamble C, Brennan G. *Working with Serious Mental Illness: a manual for clinical practice*. 2nd ed. London: Elsevier; 2006.

5 Poston JM, Hanson WE. Meta analysis of psychological assessment as a therapeutic intervention. *Psychological Assessment*. 2010; **22**: 203–12.

6 Laing RD. *The Politics of the Family and Other Essays*. London: Tavistock; 1971.

7 World Health Organization. *The ICD-10 Classification of Mental and Behavioural Disorders: clinical descriptions and diagnostic guidelines*. Geneva: World Health Organization; 1992.

8 American Psychiatric Association. *Diagnostic and Statistical Manual of Mental Disorders*. 4th ed. Text revision. Washington, DC: American Psychiatric Association; 2000.

9 Bentall RP. *Madness Explained: psychosis and human nature*. London: Penguin; 2003.

10 World Health Organization. *WHO Constitution Definition of Health*. Geneva: World Health Organization; 1984.

11 Ramachandran VS, Blakeslee S. *Phantoms in the Brain: probing the mysteries of the human mind*. New York: William Morrow and Company; 1998.

12 Adams M, Stacey-Emile G. Assessment. In: Cooper DB, editor. *Care in Mental Health–Substance Use*. London: Radcliffe Publishing; 2011.

13 National Institute of Clinical Excellence. *Guidance on Cancer Services: improving supportive and palliative care for adults with cancer. The manual*. London: NICE; 2004. www.nice.org.uk/guidance/csgsp

14 Sims A. *Symptoms in the Mind: an introduction to descriptive psychopathology.* 3rd ed. Philadelphia: Saunders; 2003.

15 Lee H. *To Kill a Mockingbird.* London: Mandarin; 1989.

16 Hall ET. *The Hidden Dimension.* New York: Doubleday; 1966.

17 Felker B, Yazel J, Short D. Mortality and medical co-morbidity among psychiatric patients: a review. *Psychiatric Services.* 1996; **47**: 1356–63.

18 Hansen V, Arnesen E, Jacobsen BK. Total mortality in people admitted to a psychiatric hospital. *British Journal of Psychiatry.* 1997; **170**: 186–90.

19 Hippisley-Cox, Fielding K, Pringle M. Depression as risk factor for ischaemic heart disease in men: population-based control study. *British Medical Journal.* 1998; **316**: 1714–19.

20 Dickey B, Normand SLT, Weiss RD, *et al.* Medical morbidity, mental illness and substance use disorders. *Psychiatric Services.* 2002; **53**: 862–7.

21 Baldwin D, Mayers A. Sexual side-effects of antidepressant and antipsychotic drugs. *Advanced Psychiatric Treatment.* 2003; **9**: 202–10.

22 Kessler RC, Chiu WT, Demler O, *et al.* Prevalence, severity, and co-morbidity of 12-month DSM-IV disorders in the National Co-morbidity Survey replication. *Archives of General Psychiatry.* 2005; **62**: 617–27.

23 Palmer BA, Pankratz VS, Bostwick JM. The lifetime risk of suicide in schizophrenia: a re-examination. *Archives of General Psychiatry.* 2005; **62**: 247–53.

24 Department of Health. *Mental Health Act 1983.* Available at: www.legislation.gov.uk/ukpga/1983/20/contents (accessed 6 March 2014).

25 Greenwald HP. Interethnic differences in pain perception. *Pain.* 1991; **44**: 57–63.

26 Riley JL, Wade JB, Myers CD, *et al.* Racial-ethnic differences in the experience of chronic pain. *Pain.* 2002; **100**: 291–8.

27 Ahmad K, Bhugra D. Depression across ethnic minority cultures: diagnostic issues. *World Cultural Psychiatry Research Review.* 2007; **2**: 47–56.

28 Sharpley M, Hutchinson G, McKenzie K, *et al.* Understanding the excess of psychosis among African-Caribbean population in England: review of current hypothesis. *British Journal of Psychiatry.* 2001; **178**: s60–s68.

29 Morris D. *Manwatching: a field guide to human behaviour.* London: Chatto, Bodley Head and Jonathan Cape; 1977.

30 Spitzer RL. The diagnostic status of homosexuality in DSM-III: a reformulation of the issues. *American Journal of Psychiatry.* 1981; **138**: 210–15.

31 Furst PT. *Flesh of the Gods: the ritual use of hallucinogens.* London: Allen & Unwin; 1972.

32 Winstock AR, Griffiths P, Stewart D. Drugs and the dance music scene: a survey of current drug use patterns among a sample of dance music enthusiasts in the UK. *Drug and Alcohol Dependence.* 2001; **64**: 9–17.

33 Bhugra D, Bhui K. Cross cultural psychiatric assessment. *Advances in Psychiatric Treatment.* 1997; **3**: 103–10.

34 Bhattacharya R, Cross S, Bhugra D. *Clinical Topics in Cultural Psychiatry.* London: Royal College of Psychiatry Publications; 2010.

35 Guarnaccia PJ, Rogler LH. Research on culture-bound syndromes: new directions. *American Journal of Psychiatry.* 1999; **156**: 1322–7.

36 Simons RC, Hughes CC, editors: *The Culture-bound Syndromes: folk illnesses of psychiatric and anthropological interest.* Dordrecht: D Reidel; 1985.

37 Banks CG. 'Culture' in culture-bound syndromes: the case of anorexia nervosa. *Social Science and Medicine.* 1992; **34**: 867–84.

38 Cooper DB. Transcultural issues and approaches. In: Wright H, Giddey M, editors. *Mental Health Nursing: from first principles to professional practice.* London: Chapman and Hall; 1993.

TO LEARN MORE

- Bentall RP. *Madness Explained: psychosis and human nature*. London: Penguin; 2003.
- International Society for the Psychological Treatment of Schizophrenias and other Psychoses (ISPS). An international organisation promoting psychotherapy and psychological treatments for people experiencing schizophrenia and other psychotic conditions. Available at: www.isps. org (accessed 6 March 2014).
- MIND. Mind helps people take control of their mental health by providing information and advice, and campaigning to promote and protect good mental health. Available at: www.mind. org.uk (accessed 6 March 2014).
- Read J, Mosher LR, Bentall RP, editors. *Models of Madness: psychological, social and biological approaches to schizophrenia*. New York: Routledge; 2004.
- Soteria Network. A network of people promoting the development of drug-free and minimum medication therapeutic medication environments for people experiencing 'psychosis' or extreme states. Available at: www.soterianetwork.org.uk/index.php (accessed 22 April 2012).
- Rudnick A, Roe D, editors. *Serious Mental Illness: person-centered approaches*. London: Radcliffe Publishing; 2011.

CULTURAL CONSIDERATIONS[12,38]

Examples of how references and beliefs can be misinterpreted through lack of knowledge of cultural issues.

➤ When a person of Pakistan origin refers to him- or herself as being 'royal', he or she is not necessarily deluded; it means simply that he or she comes from a wealthy family. This is not a grandiose delusion in cultural terms.

➤ 'The good Lord is talking to me' is an expression often used by Afro-Caribbean people of religious background. This can be misconstrued as the individual experiencing auditory hallucinations.

➤ Peoples of Asian, East Indian and African descent can have what appears to be bruising that is common among darker skinned persons. For example, what appears to be bruising on a child's body or on the individual can be 'Mongolian blue spot'. Do not jump to conclusions without adequate exploration and assessment of possible concerns.

The following list of dos and don'ts (Box 7.1) applies to all cultures. The list is not exhaustive; it can be used as a reference when working with individuals from any culture.

> **BOX 7.1** Cultural considerations – dos and don'ts[12,35]

> **Name**
> - ***Do not***:
>   - use Western titles, e.g. Mr, Miss, Ms, Mrs
>   - ask non-Christians for a Christian name.
> - ***Do***:
>   - ask for family name or first name
>   - ask what name the person prefers you use, e.g. Mr or Miss or first name
>   - use the chosen form of address

— avoid repetition in clinical notes; find out the correct name first rather than misuse several different names.

Language
* *Do not*:
  — assume that all ethnic groups speak English
  — assume that all minority ethnic groups do not speak English
  — use the family to interpret intimate questions
  — use the family to break bad news; she or he may avoid the issue if it is believed to be too stressful for the individual.
* *Do*:
  — avoid making assumptions by using accurate assessment procedures
  — use an interpreter who understands medical terminology; this will avoid stress for the interpreter, individual and family and will avoid misinterpretation.

Religion
* *Do not*:
  — generalise about the individual's or family's religion
  — mistake religious objects or symbols for jewellery.
* *Do*:
  — remember that for Buddhist, Christian, Jewish, Sikh, Hindu and Muslim people, religion may be an integral part of daily life
  — avoid incorrect assumptions; find out the different beliefs and approaches
  — record clearly and make a note of the individual's or family's wish to see or have a religious representative present
  — ask the family if the individual is not able to relay this to you
  — remember that many Eastern religions fast on certain days; pray at certain times; and wear religious objects and symbols
  — check if interventions or treatments will compromise any religious beliefs
  — inform the individual and family of any interventions or treatments, before commencing, to check religious beliefs
  — check religious observations with the individual and family
  — consult religious advisers or teachers to gain permission and/or to obtain exemption, to allow procedures to take place; ensure she or he explains this to the individual and family.

Diet
* *Do not*:
  — give Jewish or Muslim people pork or pork products.
* *Do*:
  — make sure that other meat offered to Muslim people has been religiously slaughtered by the Halal method (natural slaughter)
  — remember that not all Jewish people eat Kosher food (specially prepared to be pure)

– remember not all Muslim people eat Halal meat
– consult the individual and family about any dietary preferences
– remember that meal times are family occasions in Eastern cultures; matters relating to family are often discussed then
– remember that being taken out of a close family environment can be frightening and cause loneliness, which may in turn cause loss of appetite
– invite the family to bring food and join in meal times, if at all possible; if this is not practicable, explain why.

Personal hygiene
● *Do*:
– remember that to Sikh, Hindu and Muslim people, washing in still water is considered unclean
– supply the individual with a jug of water and bowl and/or running tap and empty washbasin to allow hands, face and body washing
– make exceptions if the individual is dependent
– remember that Muslim people use the right hand for eating and preparing food, and the left hand for self-cleaning and other procedures; anyone unable to do this because of injury or health reasons will need counselling and discussion relating to ways of surmounting this problem (it may be useful to supply plastic gloves).

Modesty
● *Do not*:
– compromise the individual's dignity and modesty.
● *Do*:
– remember that to expose the female body to a male will cause distress in certain cultures, especially if the individual is in purdah (the duration of menstruation)
– offer separate bays in mixed-bed wards or, if possible, a single room, especially if the person is in purdah
– remember that hospital gowns expose more than they cover and therefore are often unacceptable
– avoid exposure of arms and legs; add additional covering to protect modesty.

Skin and hair
● *Do*:
– remember that Afro-Caribbean people's hair may be brittle or dry; add moisturiser or oil to the scalp and comb regularly
– remember to ask the individual what she or he uses for skin moisturiser
– remember that dark-skinned people are prone to keloid scarring (hyperkeratinisation); invasive treatment will cause excessive pigmented scarring
– remember to inject or undertake invasive procedures at a site that will avoid disfigurement if possible.

Hospital procedures

- *Do not*:
  - give Jehovah's Witness people blood transfusions
  - give Muslim, Jewish and vegetarian people iron injections derived from pigs
  - give insulin of bovine origin to Hindu and Sikh people
  - give insulin of porcine origin to Jewish or Muslim people.
- *Do*:
  - give careful thought to procedures and routines before commencing them
  - remember that discussion of elimination or other intimate issues may be culturally offensive
  - approach all individuals sensitively; ensure privacy, and maintain the individual's right to self-respect
  - remember that some medications, interventions and treatments may be taboo for some religious groups
  - remember that some medications have an alcohol base which may be forbidden in some cultural groups
  - remember that individuals with alcohol problems may wish to avoid alcohol-based preparations
  - be aware of all preparations likely to contain potentially taboo or offensive ingredients.

Visiting

- *Do*:
  - remember that limiting visiting to two people may cause distress in extended family cultures
  - remember West Indian, Asian and Middle Eastern families like to visit as a family
  - remember that family may include children, uncles, aunts, grandchildren, parents and grandparents
  - compromise over visiting, and numbers of visitors per individual, if possible
  - remember that open visiting is more accommodating
  - allow the family to participate in the individual's care.

Pain myths

- *Do not*:
  - believe that people from different races have a low pain threshold; this is incorrect, for example:
  (i) Japanese people may smile or laugh when in pain, thus avoiding loss of face
  (ii) Anglo-Saxon people may be sullen and withdrawn, portraying the 'stiff-upper-lip' image
  (iii) Eastern Europeans, Greeks and Italian people express pain vocally and freely.
- *Do*:
  - remember that every individual has a different level of pain tolerance, regardless of race, colour or creed.

Death and bereavement

- ***Do not:***
  - deny a family member the right to participate in last offices, as this will increase the pain already being expressed and may slow down the grieving process.
- ***Do:***
  - involve the individual and family in care
  - remember that Eastern European cultures like to take an active part in the care of the dying relative, especially last offices
  - remember that in certain cultures, custom and practice will need to be followed if the individual is to proceed along the continuum of life following his or her earthly death
  - ensure you are fully conversant with specific cultural requirements for death, bereavement and last offices
  - negotiate to minimise anxiety and allow some participation; when the family's wishes come into conflict with hospital policies and procedures, this will assist the grieving process
  - compromise; the individual and family have only one chance to say their goodbyes.

ACKNOWLEDGEMENT

Thanks is given to the author, editors and publisher for permitting the edited reproduction of Ashcroft JR. Assessment. In: Cooper DB, Cooper J. *Palliative Care within Mental Health: principles and philosophy*. London/New York: Radcliffe Publishing; 2012. pp. 143–65.

CHAPTER 8

Pain management

Peter Athanasos, Trevor W Mitten, Rose Neild,
Charlotte de Crespigny, Lynette Cusack

CAUTIONARY NOTE

Medication of choice varies between countries. In this chapter, we use the UK model. However, the reader should take careful note that whatever their country's medication of choice, the emphasis is always on effective pain management, i.e. the right dose at the right time using the right route.

PRE-READING EXERCISE 8.1

> **Time: 15 minutes**
> - What questions could you ask a person under your care about his or her pain?
> - Have you used a pain assessment scale to assess pain?
>   - Which one did you use?
>   - Why?
>   - Is there a better one available?
> - Think of a time you, or someone close to you, were experiencing pain.
>   - What steps did you take to identify the cause of the pain and to manage it?
> - Review your answers at the end of this chapter to see if you have explored all approaches, or if you could have achieved more effective pain management.

INTRODUCTION

One of the biggest challenges facing health professionals is adequate pain management. It is generally accepted that severe pain is poorly treated in the general population. There may be a number of reasons for this.

➤ Prescribing professionals may not prescribe adequate amounts of opioids for fear of respiratory depression or cognitive and psychomotor effects, e.g. driving a car or operating machinery.

➤ The prescriber may fear the development of iatrogenic dependence (i.e. causing the person to become addicted by prescribing opioids for pain). This is a relatively rare occurrence.

➤ The prescriber may fear that the person may divert (use in a way other than prescribed or give or sell to another person) their prescription opioid drugs if given too liberally or in excess of requirement.[1]

➤ The prescriber may also have a poor understanding of the pharmacodynamics and pharmacokinetics of medication in the context of pain and prescribe ineffectively.[2]

SELF-ASSESSMENT EXERCISE 8.1

> **Time: 5 minutes**
> What would you consider to be the primary aims of pain management?

PRIMARY AIMS OF PAIN MANAGEMENT

➤ good night's sleep
➤ relief of pain at rest
➤ relief of pain on movement – although this may be more difficult to achieve.

Assessing pain

In pain management, the single most important factors are:
➤ ask the *right* questions
➤ *listen* to the answers.

The pre-requisite for good pain management is a full and comprehensive history.

An essential aid to pain assessment is the family and significant others. It is imperative that family views are sought and taken into account. The person may not wish to be seen as complaining or weak, and therefore pain may be under-reported. The response of significant others to the pain and related disability of the individual will influence the pain experience of that individual. Moreover, it is possible for pain to be 'eased' or to disappear altogether during conversation with the professional.

The individual may experience *referred* pain in one area that originates from elsewhere. Many individuals with chronic pain from a variety of causes will report multiple pains. Sufferers may experience both neuropathic and nociceptive pain simultaneously.[3] It is important to ask if the individual is experiencing different types of pain, as it is likely they will have more than one. Equally, the pain experienced might not be directly related to the primary pathology (for example, cancer). However, it is important to address all pain.

Ongoing assessment and evaluation of pain is pivotal: a continual process, not a 'one-off' exercise. It may be that as one pain is managed the individual becomes aware of another. Pain may also reappear later and/or be experienced as a different type of pain.

Assessment tools

The use of pain diaries or pain assessment tools is an important part of assessment, and gives the person a sense of control. Rating mechanisms include:

➤ visual analogue scale
➤ numerical rating scale
➤ London Hospital's Pain Chart[4] – the individual draws the pain site on a body outline.

Pain assessment in populations such as cognitively impaired older adults can be difficult to assess and this can result in poor management and outcomes.[5] Examples of assessment in this group include:
➤ Abbey pain scale[6] – a structured pain assessment scale in end-stage dementia
➤ Doloplus 2[7] – a scale for the older person with verbal communication problems.

However, whilst assessment tools have a valuable role, they are not effective in isolation and should form part of a full verbal and observational assessment.

Assessing the unconscious person

Relatives often ask whether it is possible to tell if someone unconscious is in pain. The signs can include:
➤ restlessness
➤ frowning
➤ tachycardia
➤ hypertension/autonomic instability.

This can be contrasted with the 'groaning' breathing sometimes evident in the last few hours of life, where the individual is not in pain, but has noisy respiration.

Pain awareness

Terminology is important. The person may deny pain. This may be because of adaptation to chronic pain: the individual is unable to acknowledge or verbalise its presence. Denial is a means of surviving with the pain. It is common for pain to be described as *discomfort* rather than directly to describe it as pain. By asking the individual if they have discomfort or an ache, pain may be acknowledged. This should therefore not be ignored but explored carefully with the individual and family.

Perception of pain is a very individual process, with contributions from the physical sensation of pain, personal coping styles, co-existing illnesses including depression and anxiety as well as a wealth of social and cultural factors. Even though the individuals' reports of pain are accepted as the most reliable indicator of how much pain is experienced, they may not provide necessary information to identify specific areas of pain-related disability and highlight foci for intra-/inter-disciplinary intervention planning.[8] If effective intervention in pain management is to be achieved, it needs to be acknowledged that the individual knows their own body more than anyone else, and accept that they hold the key to the problem of their pain. This information is used together with various pain assessment scales as required.

Breakthrough pain

Breakthrough pain is an increase of pain that *spikes* above a baseline of controlled pain. These episodes of pain can increase markedly, and need rapidly acting analgesia – sometimes referred to as a *rescue dose* – to reduce the pain (*see* Figure 8.1).

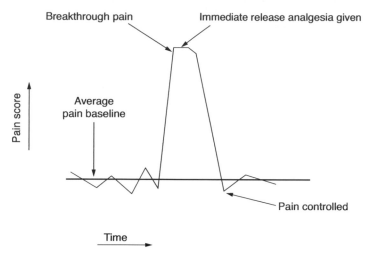

Figure 8.1 Breakthrough pain

Rapidly increasing pain

Rapid increases in pain levels may be experienced. This often occurs during the final stages of life, and is frightening for the individual and family. It often causes considerable feelings of anxiety and panic. Prompt review, a calm manner and appropriate intervention may help to allay fears and concerns. The importance of understanding that such situations can arise, and that they require prompt, effective management, cannot be over-emphasised.

Analgesia may need to be increased rapidly, especially as the situation can change within the hour. Some professionals express concern at how quickly the need for pain relief increases. This can be a source of anxiety for the professional. The need for analgesia during terminal illness is often considerably greater than the level of analgesia prescribed by the professional on a routine basis. *There is no good reason for withholding adequate analgesia.* Discussion within the intra-/inter-disciplinary team including the substance use services (e.g. alcohol and other drugs) will help to support the professional (*see* Chapter 14).

SELF-ASSESSMENT EXERCISE 8.2

Time: 5 minutes
- What non-pharmacological methods to relieve pain can you think of?
- Have you used these to relieve pain?
- If so, what relief did they provide?

Simple measures

Often the professional finds that the focus is on medication, which is perceived as a panacea for the relief of pain. Nevertheless, simple measures can often be effective. Simple measures are non-invasive, readily available and, most importantly, empower the individual, family and/or carer to feel they can do something to lessen suffering themselves. Simple measures include:

➤ pillows – careful positioning and judicious use
➤ heat therapy:
 — hot bath
 — wheat bag – check for allergies first, as some people may develop an allergic reaction to the wheat, or the bags may be impregnated with aromatherapy oils[9]
 — heat pad
➤ massage
➤ movement – changing position and simple movements can help to reduce positional pain.

KEY POINT 8.1

- Not all pain can be completely relieved.
- It is important that the individual is supported through their pain.

ANALGESIC LADDER

The World Health Organization (WHO) analgesic ladder[10] is a useful guide to prescription of the appropriate level of analgesia (*see* Figure 8.2). This progresses from Step 1, when the use of non-opioids, e.g. paracetamol and non-steroidal anti-inflammatory drugs (NSAIDs, e.g. ibuprofen) may be appropriate. If the pain remains uncontrolled, although the maximum dose has been achieved, then progression

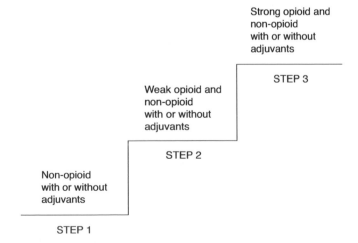

Figure 8.2 WHO Three-Step Ladder[10]

to Step 2 follows. A weak opioid, e.g. a paracetamol with codeine combination, an aspirin with codeine combination or dihydrocodeine, may be effective. These may be alternated with NSAIDs (e.g. ibuprofen) and other adjuvants as appropriate. An adjuvant (or co-analgesic) is a drug that has an independent analgesic effect or additive analgesic properties when used with opioids (e.g. NSAIDs, tramadol, ketamine, gabapentin). Step 3 drugs include the strong opioids, e.g. morphine, prescribed with or without adjuvant drugs.

KEY POINT 8.2

- Adjuvant drugs are used to complement other drugs and to maximise pain relief (*see* Figure 8.3, p. 106).
- They can be used at any step of the analgesic ladder.

A stumbling block

The main problem with prescribing analgesics is reluctance in moving from level-two to level-three drugs. Professionals, individuals and family appear concerned about morphine and describe the pain as 'not that bad yet' when faced with a choice of progression to such drugs. However, if the maximum dose of a level-two drug is achieved without effect, there is little evidence to suggest replacing this with another level-two drug. Level three is the logical progression if pain management is to be effective.

KEY POINT 8.3

- The WHO analgesic ladder is merely a guide to pain management. It is neither essential nor necessary to follow the ladder in all cases.
- For some people it may be more appropriate to prescribe Step 3 drugs immediately – hence the need for a thorough assessment of pain.

OPIOIDS IN PAIN MANAGEMENT

There are multiple liquid preparations of morphine. These are generally absorbed quickly (peak plasma concentration is 15–60 minutes),[11] and are useful for breakthrough pain, or to assess opioid need *prior* to switching to a long-acting formulation.

Oral morphine

- ➤ Strong opioid of choice for cancer.
- ➤ Regular laxative should be prescribed whenever morphine is used, as constipation almost inevitably occurs.
- ➤ Initially an anti-emetic may be needed if nausea or vomiting is a problem.
- ➤ Sedation can be a problem with large doses, though the individual does adapt to the increased dose and becomes less sedated after 3–4 days. This can recur with each dose increase.

➤ *Regular use* of morphine is much more effective than as required doses.[12]
➤ Standard strengths in the United Kingdom (UK) are:
  — 10 mg/5 mL
  — 100 mg/5 mL
➤ Oral morphine preparations may taste sharp but can be sweetened, e.g. with a little neat blackcurrant cordial.

Oral morphine – use of quick-acting preparations

KEY POINT 8.4

- Commence morphine using a quick-acting liquid or tablet before switching to sustained-release morphine.
- Enable rapid titration to the therapeutic level.
- Oral rescue doses of liquid morphine can be offered every 30 minutes in extreme cases.[13]

Sublingual

The administration of sublingual morphine can be used in terminal stages. It may be considered where remote location or lack of other medications precludes other alternatives. In the UK, there is a tablet form of quick-release morphine called Sevredol, available as 10 mg, 20 mg and 50 mg.

Breakthrough pain

Oral doses for breakthrough pain can be offered every 60 minutes if needed.[14] The rescue dose for breakthrough pain is one-third of the 12-hourly dose of sustained-release morphine. It is important to review the effect of the morphine and the pain regularly. The dose should be increased as appropriate, taking into account all of the rescue doses taken within a 24-hour period. If additional doses are required several times during the day, consider whether the regular dose needs to be increased.[3]

KEY POINT 8.5

When pain is problematic at night, and wakes the person, increase the dose of oral morphine at bedtime.

In the UK, morphine sulphate tablets (MST), in a sustained-release formulation, are available in 5 mg, 10 mg, 15 mg, 30 mg, 60 mg, 100 mg and 200 mg strengths, and are suitable for twice-daily administration. If pain is not relieved by 90% after 24 hours, increase the dose,[3] e.g. from:
➤ 5 to 10 mg
➤ 10 to 15 mg
➤ 20 to 30 mg.

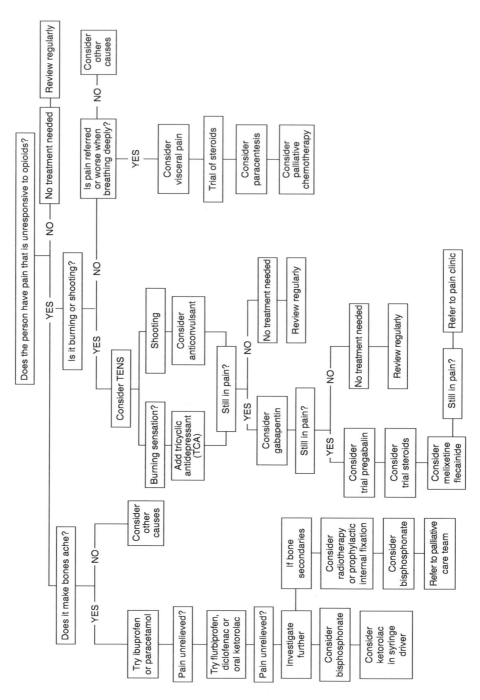

Figure 8.3 Flow chart for opioid-unresponsive pain

In addition, consider adjuvant drugs when administering strong opioids (NSAIDs, tramadol, ketorolac, ketamine – *see* Figure 8.3).

KEY POINT 8.6

Different types of pain, e.g. bone or nerve pain, respond to different types of medication. We need to try different opioids and different adjuvants.

Opioid preparations

There are several long- and short-acting opioid preparations summarised in Table 8.1.

TABLE 8.1 Long- and short-acting opioid preparations

Drug	Starting dose	Indications for use
Fentanyl transmucosal-lozenge on a stick (Actiq)	200 micrograms repeated after 15 minutes if pain unrelieved	For rapid relief of incident or breakthrough pain. Good for those unable to take oral medication.
Fentanyl Transdermal Therapeutic System (TTS) (fentanyl patch)	25 micrograms every 72 hours	Stable severe pain.
Hydromorphone	4 mg 12-hourly	Can be opened and sprinkled onto soft, cold food.
Methadone	Specialist advice is needed pre-prescription	Used for severe pain, intractable cough and opioid rotation.
		It has a long half-life in the body (i.e. it takes a long time to be broken down), and can accumulate to toxic levels (*seek specialist advice*). May be beneficial for neuropathic pain. For cough a dose of 2–4 mg at night or twice daily may help.
Morcap (UK) capsules of morphine	20 mg once a day (licensed for 12-hourly administration)	This is a capsule form of morphine (available in the UK) that can be opened and sprinkled onto food.
MST continuous suspension (prolonged release granules of morphine)	10–30 mg twice a day for opioid-naïve persons or those previously on weak opioids	MST suspension is a sachet of powder which, when mixed with water, forms a suspension of prolonged-release granules of morphine that the person drinks (available in the UK). This is useful if swallowing tablets is a problem. It can also be syringed down a gastrostomy tube. It is available in a variety of doses up to 200 mg sachet but is difficult to mix without forming lumps. To ensure even distribution of the mix use 10–20 mL of very hot water as the base, and sprinkle the powder on slowly whilst stirring gently. Ensure the mix is cool before administration.

(*continued*)

Drug	Starting dose	Indications for use
MXL (sustained-release morphine)	30 mg once a day	This is a once-daily capsule preparation of sustained-release morphine (UK).
Oramorph (oral morphine sulphate)	10–30 mg 4-hourly as needed	Useful for breakthrough pain. Absorbed quickly.
Oxycodone	30 mg suppository 8-hourly	Useful for people who are unable to tolerate oral medication. This is given as a suppository, providing 6–8 hours of relief. Useful if unable to take orally and a syringe driver is inappropriate.
Oxycodone	10 mg oral twice daily	Lasts 12 hours.
OxyNorm (oxycodone capsules and liquid)	Capsules 5 mg Liquid 5 mg/5 ml	Both immediate-release, last 4–6 hours.
Sevredol (immediate release morphine tablet)	10–30 mg 4-hourly	Used for breakthrough pain. Immediate release morphine in tablet form.

Prescribing consideration

Consideration must be given to possible adverse effects related to opioid use (*see* Table 8.2). These may include:

➤ **possible toxic effects** – respiratory depression, prolonged QTC (a measure of the time between the start of the Q *wave* and the end of the T *wave* in the heart's electrical cycle) interval

➤ **intolerable side effects** – constipation, nausea, vomiting, sedation – which may outweigh the benefits

TABLE 8.2 Morphine side effects

Side effect	Treatment
Constipation	Laxatives, e.g.: • Co-danthramer (dantron, poloxamer 188) • senna • docusate.
Nausea/ vomiting	Anti-emetics: • cyclizine (caution: significant interaction with methadone if used) • haloperidol • metoclopramide. *Often passes after a few days so need to review*
Drowsiness	None: passes after a few days but may recur temporarily after dose increase.
Bad dreams/ hallucinations	• infrequent. Need to assess for opioid toxicity • reduce dose • add antipsychotic, e.g. haloperidol 1.5 mg three times daily • switch to different strong opioids (e.g. methadone, fentanyl etc)

➤ **renal failure** – accumulation of morphine metabolites may lead to increased sedation and respiratory depression – may need to rotate to an opioid that is less effected by renal failure (such as methadone)[15]

➤ **fear of morphine** – and an unwillingness to take the drug. This may be fear of the side effects of morphine or fear of 'becoming addicted'. Please *see* 'Iatrogenic dependency' below. Alternative opioids may elicit compliance.

Diamorphine profile (heroin)

➤ Chemically, diamorphine consists of two morphine molecules locked together.
➤ It is the preferred drug of choice for use in a syringe driver for subcutaneous infusion.
➤ It has a much higher solubility in solutions.
➤ It is twice as potent as morphine when administered by subcutaneous injection.[16]

OxyContin – prolonged release oxycodone hydrochloride

A long-acting 12-hourly oxycodone tablet (OxyContin). Ten mg oral OxyContin is approximately equivalent to 20 mg oral morphine.[17] Twelve-hourly strengths range from 5–120 mg.

An immediate-relief quick-acting liquid or tablet form (OxyNorm) is available.[17] There is also a rectal preparation – oxycodone suppositories.

Fentanyl

The transdermal patch (Durogesic DTrans, fentanyl) is a clear sticky patch, applied to the skin, that normally lasts three days. Durogesic DTrans is smaller and adheres better than previous patches. Fentanyl patches may cause less constipation and the daytime somnolence caused by morphine.[18] Transdermal patches in the UK are in five strengths:

1 12 microgram
2 25 microgram
3 50 microgram
4 75 microgram
5 100 microgram.

The patch will provide good pain relief, and seem less intrusive than the subcutaneous route. If a patch is already in place, it is unwise to rotate to another strong opioid at the end-of-life[19] unless pain is increasing, as the crossover period may lead to pain breakthrough. It is best to continue with the same patch.

Essential knowledge for fentanyl patch preparation

➤ Fentanyl can take from 12 to 24 hours to achieve maximum blood concentration.[12]
➤ If the person is currently receiving morphine sulphate tablets (MST), the fentanyl patch is applied with the last oral dose of MST.[20]
➤ Fentanyl patches are not suitable if pain is escalating rapidly, due to slow absorption rate.

➤ It is essential that individuals with fentanyl patches are prescribed quick-release opioids for breakthrough pain:
   — this must be given in the correct dose for the patch size
   — the dose should be increased whenever the patch size is increased.
➤ Some reports have indicated that the fentanyl patch only lasts for 2 days.[21] *The normal application period is 3 days.* If pain control is maximised at 2 days but decreases on day 3, the patch can be changed on the second day.
➤ Continual review of pain is pivotal.
➤ Counselling is essential for the individual and family throughout.
➤ Verbal and written guidance about the application of the patch is essential.
➤ Careful explanation of the potential side effects will ease anxiety and aid compliance.
➤ People *do* find the patches advantageous as:
   — the need for oral medication is reduced
   — comfort is increased
   — the daily reminders relating to health may be decreased.
➤ The normal starting dose is a 12–25 microgram patch. If the person is converting from 4-hourly oral morphine to fentanyl, the morphine should be *continued for 12 hours* while the blood concentration achieves maximum saturation.
➤ If the person wearing the fentanyl patch is experiencing breakthrough pain, *divide the fentanyl patch by 5* (Patch/5) to give the dose in milligrams of diamorphine administered subcutaneously.[22] This will aid management of breakthrough pain.

Adverse effects

A small number of people experience adverse effects in the first 24 hours when switching from morphine to fentanyl patches.[20] These can include:
➤ sweating
➤ diarrhoea
➤ bowel cramps
➤ nausea
➤ restlessness.

Treatment

These adverse effects are the consequence of opioid withdrawal caused by rapid decreases in opioid dose during the changeover period. One or two doses of oral morphine will give quick release of adverse effects.

Other fentanyl preparations

➤ trans-mucosal lozenge on a stick – for rapid reduction of breakthrough pain[23]
➤ intravenous injection (alfentanyl) – good in renal failure
➤ subcutaneous via syringe driver (alfentanyl) – for morphine intolerance.

Topical opioids

Topical opioids in a carrier gel (intrasite or metronidazole) for wound pain can be beneficial.[24–26] Topical opioids:

➤ can be helpful for a wound, e.g. pressure ulcer
➤ can be effective co-jointly with systemic opioids.[27]

One regime is 1 mg of diamorphine to 1 mg of intrasite gel applied once daily.[28] Another is in the use of diamorphine and instillagel local anaesthetic gel, or with KY Jelly.[29]

KEY POINT 8.7

● Fear of seeing the wound may heighten perceived pain.[26]
● Minimise the person's exposure to seeing the wound during dressing changes – unless otherwise requested by the person.

Does adding a second opioid improve pain relief?

Inadequate pain management, with escalating opioid doses, in the presence of dose-limiting toxic effects, including:

➤ hallucinations
➤ confusion
➤ hyperalgesia
➤ myoclonus (brief involuntary twitching of muscles or group of muscles)
➤ sedation
➤ nausea

may be a problem in some cases. When the person requires increasing doses of a strong analgesic, benefit may be obtained from using two opioids or by combining an opioid with a non-opioid adjuvant such as tramadol, ketamine, a gabapentanoid or a non-steroidal anti-inflammatory drug (NSAID).[30]

In this situation, the combination of two different opioids or a non-opioid adjuvant analgesic with an opioid may be advantageous for three reasons:

1 it may provide a multimodal coverage of a broad spectrum of pain
2 it may enable the individual agents to act in a greater than additive (synergistic) fashion
3 it may lower doses of each individual analgesic and may result in a lower incidence of individual adverse events.[30]

Opioid-unresponsive pain

Pains not fully responsive to opioids include:

➤ **musculoskeletal** – bone pain. Typical description:
  – aching joints – sometimes described as toothache; a pressure and/or heaviness in the bone – may be experienced in the back or hip. This is often worse on movement

➤ **neurogenic** – nerve pain. Typical description:
  — stabbing
  — shooting
  — burning
  — pins and needles
  — increased sensitivity of skin
  — change in sensation.

KEY POINT 8.8

Careful and attentive listening to the description of the pain provides vital information relating to pain type.

Musculoskeletal – bone pain

Bone pain may arise for a variety of reasons, including:
➤ osteoarthritis
➤ pathological fracture
➤ bone metastases.

The first-line drugs of choice are non-steroidal anti-inflammatory drugs (NSAIDs). Because of the anti-inflammatory effect, NSAIDs are useful for metastatic bone and soft tissue pains. They can be used with strong opioids[3] (*see* Table 8.3).

TABLE 8.3 Anti-inflammatory drugs

Drug	Dose
Aspirin	600 mg four times a day
Ibuprofen	200–600 mg three times a day or brufen retard (ibuprofen sustained-release) two tablets daily (800 mg)
Flurbiprofen (Froben)	• 50 mg three times daily • 100 mg three times daily
Diclofenac (Voltarol)	• oral – 50 mg three times daily • oral – 75 mg twice daily • suppositories 100 mg
Keterolac (Toradol)	• oral – 10 mg three times daily • subcutaneous infusion – 60–120 mg over 24 hours
Piroxicam (Feldene)	• oral – 20 mg once daily
Feldene melt	• dissolve on tongue

Essential knowledge for NSAID preparations

➤ NSAIDs help to control bone pain.
➤ It is worth rotating to different non-steroidal drugs if one particular drug does not work.[31]
➤ Ketorolac is a NSAID which is available in tablet form (10 mg three times daily/ four times daily)[17] or by intravenous or subcutaneous injection.[32]

> Administration via a syringe driver is beneficial if other oral NSAIDs have failed.[33] This can be attributed to ketorolac's dual anti-inflammatory and analgesic effect.[34] The improved absorption via the parenteral route also plays a role.

> NSAIDs may cause gastric irritation. Thus a gastro-protective should be considered (proton pump inhibitors – which reduce acid in the stomach, e.g. omeprazole) and H_2 antagonists (block the action of histamine and also reduce acid in the stomach, e.g. ranitidine).[35]

SELF-ASSESSMENT EXERCISE 8.3

Time: 15 minutes
- The individual in your care says the pain is burning and continuous in nature.
- What type of pain do you think this might indicate?
- What drug treatment might be prescribed for nerve pain?
- What are the Three Steps in the WHO analgesic ladder?
- List three non-pharmacological treatments that may help to relieve pain.
- Identify three non-verbal indicators that the person may be in pain.
- What are the common side effects of morphine?
- When may fentanyl patches be indicated?

Bisphosphonates

The use of bisphosphonates in cases of bone pain is encouraging.[36] Even when individuals have a normal calcium level,[37] treatment with a bisphosphonate, e.g. – most used in the UK – pamidronate 60–90 mg intravenous (IV) every 4–6 weeks, can markedly reduce bone metastases pain. A once-a-day preparation of bisphosphonate tablet – ibandronate (Bondronat)[38,39] – eliminates the need for hospitalisation for an infusion.

Radiotherapy

> Radiation can reduce pain in 90% of people experiencing bone pain.[40]
> Radiotherapy can be helpful in reducing pain from bone metastases.
> A single dose is often all that is required for treatment.

Strontium

> Injections of strontium 89 (Metastron™) for the relief of metastatic bone pain is indicated for people with prostate or breast cancer.[41]
> Strontium follows the pathway of calcium, delivering local radiotherapy to the site of bone metastases.

Neurogenic – nerve pain

Nerve pain often follows nerve pathways, e.g. the facial nerve (trigeminal neuralgia) or thoracic nerve (shingles). It is not fully controlled by opioids,[42] but often responds well to antidepressant medication (e.g. amitriptyline, venlafaxine – particularly if the sensation is *burning*). Alternatively, anti-epileptic medication, e.g. gabapentin,[43] pregabalin[44] or carbamazepine, may be considered (*see* Table 8.4).

TABLE 8.4 Drug management of neurogenic pain

Drug	Dosage/side effects
Amitriptyline	• 10–75 mg nocte • can cause dry mouth, blurred vision, sedation
Venlafaxine	• 37.5 mg twice daily • increase to 75 mg after one week if necessary • can cause dizziness, dry mouth, insomnia, constipation
Sertraline	• 50–150 mg once daily in the morning • nausea a problem initially. Also diarrhoea, restlessness, headache
Gabapentin	• 100–600 mg three times daily – slowly titrated. *NOTE: seek advice – even if experienced* • can cause dizziness, sedation, nausea, blurred vision
Pregabalin	• 75–300 mg twice daily • can cause dizziness, sedation, peripheral oedema

Other treatments for nerve pain

➤ **Epidural/intrathecal injection** – Epidural analgesia is directed into the epidural space of the spinal cord. The epidural space is inside the bony spinal canal but outside the dura mater membrane. Intrathecal analgesia is directed into the space under the arachnoid membrane of the spinal cord or brain
➤ **Coeliac plexus block** – The coeliac plexus is also known as the solar plexus and is a complex of nerves in the abdomen. It is the injection of local anaesthetic onto these nerves for control of pain
➤ **Chemical nerve destruction** – With phenol (also known as carbolic acid), a strong neurotoxin that can destroy nerves.
➤ **Surgical nerve destruction** (e.g. cordotomy).

The flow chart (Figure 8.3) on opioid-unresponsive pain indicates considerations and actions for addressing these types of pain.

Steroids in pain management

The use of steroids in pain management needs to be weighed against the side effects. However, steroids can be effective if used appropriately. Steroids are indicated in the following:[20]
➤ raised intra-cranial pressure
➤ spinal cord compression
➤ bone pain
➤ liver capsule stretch (enlargement of the liver due to liver cancer).

Steroid use in symptom palliation

➤ reduces cerebral oedema in cerebral tumours/secondaries

➤ lowers raised intra-cranial pressure
➤ stimulates appetite
➤ provides euphoria and energy for special event, e.g. a wedding
➤ reduces liver capsule pain by decreasing swelling
➤ reduces nerve pain by relieving nerve compression or irritation.

Prescribing and administering steroids

Dexamethasone:
➤ is often the steroid of choice
➤ is approximately seven times more potent than prednisolone,[20] therefore fewer tablets are needed
➤ crosses the blood–brain barrier and is useful for people with cerebral tumours
➤ tablets can be crushed and made into a suspension with warm water, for ease of swallowing
➤ supplied as a sugar-free solution (Dexsol).[45]

To prevent dyspepsia/ulcers a proton pump inhibitor (PPI), e.g. omeprazole, or H_2 antagonist, e.g. ranitidine, helps protect the stomach.

Steroid adverse effects

➤ gastric irritation or ulceration
➤ water retention
➤ fluid imbalance
➤ immunosuppression
➤ steroid psychosis
➤ oral candidiasis
➤ insomnia
➤ thinning of the skin
➤ hypertension
➤ steroid-induced diabetes
➤ osteoporosis
➤ myopathy.

KEY POINT 8.9

- Steroids given four times a day can cause nocturnal insomnia.
- Once or twice a day (morning and lunchtime) administration is preferable.[46]

Visceral pain

Visceral pain – i.e. pain from any internal organs, especially within the abdomen – can be:
➤ worse on taking a deep breath
➤ an excruciating pain – when an organ cannot swell to accommodate a tumour due to the presence of inflexible viscera containing the organ.

The most common example is liver pain due to metastases causing liver capsule stretch, i.e. swollen liver. This is why in physical examinations the liver is palpated. Treatment is usually with morphine and steroids (dexamethasone 4–8 mg/day[20]), to reduce peri-tumour oedema. Palliative radiotherapy or chemotherapy may also be indicated.

Non-pharmacological management of pain

Transcutaneous electrical nerve stimulation (TENS)

The use of transcutaneous electrical nerve stimulation (TENS) machines has been found to be beneficial. A total of 47% of people report a 50% reduction in pain intensity after treatment.[47] TENS works by blocking the transmission of painful stimuli (referred to as the gate theory) by increasing activity in the large 'A' fibres, which block activity in the smaller pain fibres. There is a concomitant release of endorphins. It is important to read – and understand – the instructions of use prior to using a TENS machine.[47]

Psychological approaches

Pain can be:
- physical
- emotional/psychological
- spiritual
- social

… together, these are referred to as *total pain*.[48]

Anxiety

Recognition that anxiety can increase the intensity of pain is essential and pivotal to any intervention.[49] The individual and family need continuous assessment and restructuring of care as identified. Some people may benefit from counselling with regard to issues such as family problems, existential or spiritual needs in addition to analgesia (*see* Chapters 5, 7).

Hope and coping strategies

Hope and coping strategies (e.g. distraction therapy, visualisation and imagery)[50] empower the individual and enable better skills.

Relaxation and visualisation

Relaxation and visualisation can benefit the individual and family by:
- promoting sleep
- promoting management of stress and pain
- reducing anxiety and depression.[51]

Pain and/or fear can cause tension, restlessness, poor concentration and agitation. Relaxation, defined as a 'state of freedom from both anxiety and skeletal muscle tension' is helpful.[50] Simple breathing exercises can promote relaxation and may be described during counselling.

Other pain management strategies

- ➤ physiotherapy
- ➤ massage
- ➤ osteopathy
- ➤ spiritual healing.
- ➤ aromatherapy
- ➤ hypnotherapy
- ➤ acupuncture

Sometimes it is necessary to use a combination of techniques and/or relaxation in conjunction with other complementary therapies to provide an effective intervention. The decision on what is best is often trial and error and based on the individual's or the family's experience and wishes.

PAIN MANAGEMENT, SERIOUS AND ENDURING MENTAL HEALTH AND SERIOUS AND ENDURING SUBSTANCE USE

Within the concept of palliative care for the individual experiencing serious and enduring mental health problems, it is important that we consider the needs of the individual co-experiencing serious and enduring substance use problems (*see* Chapter 14). The chapter continues by examining the specific and essential needs of this population of individuals.

Pain management in the opioid-maintained population

People maintained on opioids, both for the treatment of opioid dependence (addiction) and for the treatment of chronic pain, who present to clinics and general wards with acute pain conditions, are a particular challenge.[52] These people may present with a range of medical or surgical problems causing acute pain, including serious illnesses, injuries and infectious diseases (e.g. hepatitis or human immunodeficiency virus – HIV). Acute pain management following surgery or due to trauma for these people may be especially problematic. In general, these individuals experience a greater sensitivity to pain and a cross-tolerance to analgesic effects of opioids as a result of their opioid dependence. This complicates treatment considerably.

There are three complications to pain management in this population:

1 **misunderstandings** – regarding the management of acute and chronic pain
2 **opioid tolerance** – with opioid use, opioid tolerance develops and people require more drug to maintain the same effect
3 **hyperalgesia** – with the use of opioids, there may be the paradoxical development of greater pain sensitivity.[53]

SELF-ASSESSMENT EXERCISE 8.4 (*SEE* ANSWERS ON PP. 133–4)

> **Time: 30 minutes**
> Read the following case scenario carefully then answer the questions. All names are fictitious.

Case Study – Lisa

Lisa (38) has a long-standing history of amphetamine and heroin dependence. She has been on methadone maintenance treatment for the last three years. She fell last night and fractured her forearm on a coffee table. She was admitted to the hospital. In the morning, she began to become agitated and demanded her 150 mg of methadone she claims she has daily. However, her urine drug screen has come back negative for methadone but positive for amphetamines. Lisa is scheduled for surgery on her arm later on that day.

Case questions

➤ Why might Lisa have become agitated and demanded methadone?
➤ What further information do you need and where might you find it?
➤ What should your approach to her pain relief be?
➤ How would you discuss your observations and further assess Lisa?

Common misconceptions

Many misconceptions around pain management and opioid dependence arise due to common stereotypes associated with dependence. This stereotyping can lead to inappropriate or suboptimal pain management. For example, it is important to consider that physical dependence and tolerance are typical and predictable consequences of regular frequent opioid exposure. People who use opioids for chronic pain management or treatment of opioid dependence often become tolerant to relatively high doses of opioids and require even higher doses for acute severe pain. They may require as much as 2.5–3 times the analgesic dose of non-tolerant individuals.[54,55] Similarly, people who are maintained on opioids for any reason become physically dependent; if their dose is abruptly ceased they are likely to go into withdrawal. Tolerance and hyperalgesia may occur regardless of the indication for commencing regular opioid dosing.[56] Opioid and other withdrawal syndromes may significantly worsen the experience of pain and may further complicate adequate pain management.

The physical conditions of tolerance and withdrawal do not in themselves indicate psychological dependence or problematic drug use. Definitions help to clarify the relationship between physical tolerance, dependence and pain management. Ranges of definitions are described below. Some general principles and a number of common misconceptions follow these. Specific guidelines are then described.

DEFINITIONS
Dependence
Physical dependence

Physical dependence occurs when the central nervous system (CNS) has been continually exposed to a drug and upon cessation of the drug, the CNS goes into withdrawal. A rule of thumb is that the withdrawal syndrome will be the opposite of the drug's effects on the individual. For example, one of the withdrawal symptoms from a stimulant such as methamphetamine will be feelings of fatigue and possibly extended sleep. Withdrawal symptoms from a depressant such as alcohol or opioids will include agitation, sleep disruption and anxiety.

Psychological dependence

Psychological dependence is when someone has been continually exposed to a drug and upon cessation of the drug, experiences psychological withdrawal. The person desires the drug and is preoccupied with thoughts of acquiring the drug. It may or may not be accompanied by the physical signs of withdrawal. Another definition (as well as another way to describe addiction) is the compulsion to use a drug despite knowledge that it is harmful. This process may occur with other non-drug forms of psychological dependence such as gambling or shopping.

Iatrogenic dependency

Iatrogenic dependency is where a person is treated with analgesics for a legitimate pain condition and consequently develops a dependency. People suffering from painful conditions often express concern about this. They may state 'I need pain relief, but I don't want to become addicted' or even deliberately under-report their pain. However, iatrogenic dependency is uncommon following a single surgical procedure.

In some situations, iatrogenic dependence is more likely to occur. For example, an automobile accident may result in multiple traumas for a person. The person may be required to undergo a number of surgical procedures, potentially resulting in a series of recovery periods with inadequately managed pain.

The prospect of successive undermanaged pain episodes can be extremely stressful. It is more likely that the stress associated with the anticipation of undermanaged pain will be a trigger for the development of dependence than the effective use of opioids for pain management.

Pseudo-psychological dependence

KEY POINT 8.10

Pseudo-psychological dependence, in the context of pain management, is where a person appears to be drug seeking but is merely trying to ensure adequate pain relief.

The person may exhibit extremely inappropriate behaviour in their attempts to manage their pain.

They may be:

➤ involved in illegal activity such as buying opioids on the black market
➤ 'doctor shopping'
➤ displaying aggression
➤ stockpiling large amounts of opioids
➤ going to extreme lengths to manipulate professionals and friends to obtain opioids.

Psychological or pseudo-psychological dependence?

The differentiation between psychological dependence and pseudo-psychological dependence can be difficult for the professional.

With adequate pain management these aberrant behaviours should cease and the behaviour be considered pseudo-psychological dependence. If adequate pain management is forthcoming and these behaviours do not cease, then it is likely to be psychological dependence. The confounding factor is the difficulty in ascertaining if adequate pain management is being provided.[53] Failure to provide adequate pain management may increase the likelihood of progression to psychological dependence.[57]

Tolerance

Physical tolerance

Physical tolerance occurs when progressively larger amounts of the drug are required to get the same effect. Alternatively, if the amount of drug consumed remains constant, the effect of the drug diminishes. The development of physical tolerance by people on long-term opioid therapy is the central problem for effective pain management for this population. In spite of being maintained on relatively large amounts of opioids, individuals require even larger amounts of opioids for analgesic effect. Effective pain management starts by administering the dose usually required for an opioid-naïve individual, and then titrating doses upwards until adequate pain relief is achieved. Analgesics should not be withheld unless the person is becoming over-sedated or experiencing depressed respiration.

Psychological tolerance

Psychological tolerance is when progressively larger amounts of the drug or addictive activity are required to get the same psychological effect. The person has got 'used to' the drug, the behaviour or the feelings experienced. For example, if the person has a gambling problem, they may feel the need to gamble more and more to derive the same sense of satisfaction they initially felt. This may occur without physiological changes.

A person's desired psychological effect from their drug of choice may be quite different from the prescriber's intended target therapeutic effect. Some people prefer to tolerate seemingly large amounts of pain with little analgesia. Others prefer to be sedated, thus feeling the smallest amount of discomfort. Just as the physiological perception of pain may differ between individuals, there is also a significant interpersonal variation in the psychological perception of pain. This is an important factor in a person's psychological tolerance.

Differential development of tolerance

Tolerance develops more rapidly to such effects as:

➤ analgesia
➤ sedation
➤ vomiting
➤ euphoria
➤ nausea
➤ respiratory depression.

Interestingly, it develops slowly or not at all to miosis ('pinning' of the pupils) and constipation. Those maintained on methadone and buprenorphine may complain of constipation for years after commencing treatment. It is important to remember that opioid tolerance develops to the desired effects (e.g. analgesia and euphoria) as well as the undesired effects (e.g. opioid-related sedation and nausea).

Cross-tolerance

Tolerance to one opioid makes a person cross-tolerant to another opioid. It is the mechanism by which opioid substitution works. People are given long-acting methadone or buprenorphine because it stops the withdrawal syndrome associated with a shorter-acting opioid such as heroin. Similarly benzodiazepines are administered to alcohol-dependent people to stop them going into withdrawal (alcohol and benzodiazepines act at the same receptors and so cross-tolerance occurs).

Pseudo-tolerance

Pseudo-tolerance in the context of acute pain management is where a person's level of use of a drug increases and they require an increased amount of opioid, but it is not due to the development of analgesic tolerance.

It could be due to:
➤ drug interaction – if the person starts taking a different drug, the original drug may not be as effective
➤ progression of the disease or the development of a new disease
➤ increase in physical activity.

Hyperalgesia

KEY POINT 8.11

Pain is important for human functioning.

Pain signals to the brain that certain behaviour may cause injury. During opioid maintenance, there is a relatively large amount of opioid being circulated around the body, providing analgesia. The body, in an effort to provide homeostatic balance, becomes more sensitive to pain. It 'counterbalances' the analgesic effect of the opioid to maintain responsiveness to pain. Unfortunately, it commonly sensitises more than required and people maintained on opioids become more sensitive to pain, even those with high plasma opioid concentrations, compared to opioid-naïve people.

This may contribute to the development of opioid tolerance. As the body becomes more sensitive to pain, it requires more opioid to achieve a pain-free state. As stated, it is the primary complicating factor in the pain management of opioid-dependent people.

GENERAL PRINCIPLES

> **KEY POINT 8.12**
>
> There are misconceptions around the use of opioids, pain and dependence. It is crucial that professionals have a good understanding of these general principles.

Maintenance opioids do not provide analgesia

There are three main factors preventing maintenance opioids from providing analgesia.

1 Methadone and buprenorphine have an analgesic duration of action of approximately 4–8 hours. Yet these drugs are administered and provide protection from withdrawal for 24–48 hours. Therefore, the period of pain relief is relatively small relative to dosing periods.

2 Tolerance develops very rapidly to the analgesic effects of opioids when maintained for a period of time. The person becomes tolerant to both large amounts of methadone or buprenorphine but is also cross-tolerant to the analgesic effects of other opioids.

3 The development of hyperalgesia.[53]

Adding opioids does not cause respiratory and CNS depression

Like analgesia, tolerance to the respiratory and CNS depression effects develops quickly. For example, as the pain increases for people with carcinomas, and opioid doses are increased in consequence, there is generally no increase in respiratory and CNS depression in doses adequate to achieve pain control.

> **KEY POINT 8.13**
>
> Pain is a natural antagonist to opioid-induced respiratory and CNS depression.

Seeking relief from pain is not the same as drug seeking

> **KEY POINT 8.14**
>
> Seeking relief from pain is different from drug seeking.

A careful clinical assessment for the objective evidence of pain will decrease the chance of manipulation by a drug-seeking person and also support the administration of opioid analgesics in a person with a history of drug dependence.

Professionals often perceive opioid-dependent people with pain issues to be demanding and manipulative. In turn, opioid-dependent people, often due to a history of discrimination and inadequate pain relief, may:

➤ become distrustful of the medical community and concerned about being stigmatised

➤ fear that their pain will be undertreated or that their opioid maintenance dose will be altered or discontinued

➤ act inappropriately to get opioids but only be suffering from unrelieved pain (pseudo-psychological dependence)

➤ have good pain relief but be fearful of the re-emergence of pain

➤ fear withdrawal symptoms should their pain relief be discontinued

➤ fear a reduction in the current effective doses of opioid analgesics.

Major health effects of unrelieved pain

KEY POINT 8.15

Major health implications are associated with unmanaged pain.

There are major health implications associated with unmanaged pain:

➤ physical stasis (bedsores, foot droop, etc.)

➤ prolonged post-operative recoveries

➤ clinical depression

➤ cardiovascular stress

➤ increased tumour growth

➤ relapse or exacerbation of dependence issues.

KEY POINT 8.16

It is critical for pain to be well managed to achieve optimal overall health.

Factors affecting the pain experience

The pain experience of people maintained on opioids with chronic pain is not simply augmented by opioid-induced hyperalgesia. It is also exacerbated by subtle withdrawal syndromes. It may also be influenced by intoxication with related sympathetic arousal and muscle tension. Sleep disturbance, mood changes and functional changes (associated with a comorbid condition such as hepatitis C) may also affect the pain experience.[53,58]

Identifying and treating co-occurring conditions which affect the perception of pain and, therefore, the successful management of the pain is of paramount importance. Important examples of frequently comorbid conditions are depression and anxiety. Both may significantly complicate the treatment of pain and dependence, but may be responsive to a range of treatments.

The dangers associated with unrestricted opioid dosing

The answer is not as simple as dosing without restriction in an effort to produce pain relief. While there are dangers with unmanaged pain, there are dangers with unrestricted opioid dosing. While opioids theoretically have no maximum ceiling, hyperalgesia (as stated), neuroendocrinological (hormone) dysfunction and possibly immunosuppression (decreased functioning of the immune system) may occur at high doses. Respiratory depression can present difficulties in spite of tolerance (especially if the person is on other medication or consumes alcohol or another central nervous system depressant). Sedation can interfere with daily function and the processes of driving and safety around the home, and care of dependents may be affected with lethal consequences. It has also been suggested that repeated dose escalations lack incremental benefit at higher doses (e.g. more than 200 mg of morphine daily or equivalent).[1]

SPECIFIC PAIN MANAGEMENT GUIDELINES FOR OPIOID-TOLERANT PEOPLE

People with active dependency

Build trust

➤ Openly acknowledge history of dependency, and allow people to discuss fears about how this may affect pain management and treatment by the professionals.
➤ Reassure people that their history of dependency problems will not prevent adequate pain management.
➤ Respect and believe the person's report of pain.
➤ Reassure the person that professionals are committed to assertively providing effective pain relief.
➤ Aggressively treat acute pain; treatment for dependency issues is not the priority during the acute pain period.

Professional education

➤ Prescription of opioids to a person with a known dependency problem for the management of pain is not illegal or unethical.
➤ People with a dependency problem may be relatively pain-intolerant.
➤ Detoxification is an ineffective short-term treatment for a dependency problem and inappropriate in the presence of pain.

Broaden the treatment plan

➤ With the person, develop a treatment contract for opioid analgesia.
➤ Request consultation from a substance use medicine specialist.
➤ Carefully document treatment plan, including analgesic use, response and regular reviews of efficacy of current plan.

Knowledgeably administer opioids

➤ Utilise non-pharmacologic and non-opioid analgesic alternatives (as discussed earlier).
➤ Consider patient-controlled analgesia which may decrease total opioid requirements and the drug-seeking behaviours.
➤ Choose long-acting opioids (e.g. slow-release morphine sulphate; slow-release oxycodone) with gradual onset of action and lower street value, administered

under continuous scheduled dosing orders (e.g. four times a day – q.i.d.) rather than as-needed orders (p.r.n.).

➤ Opioid cross-tolerance and the person's increased pain sensitivity will often necessitate higher opioid analgesic doses administered at shorter intervals.

KEY POINT 8.17

If physically maintained on an agonist (e.g. methadone), *do not* administer a mixed opioid agonist/antagonist (e.g. buprenorphine) – withdrawal may be precipitated.[53]

Individuals on opioid maintenance therapy

➤ Continue the usual dose of methadone or buprenorphine (or equivalent).

➤ Use short-acting opioid analgesics and titrate to effect (e.g. morphine, codeine, oxycodone).

➤ Contact methadone or buprenorphine maintenance clinic or prescribing physician:
   — notify them of admission, discharge and confirm the time and amount of last maintenance dose
   — notify them of any medications such as opioids or benzodiazepines given to the person during hospitalisation because they may show up on routine urine drug screening
   — notify them of any short-term analgesia (opioid or otherwise) provided on discharge.[53]

Individuals currently abstinent

Build trust

➤ Openly acknowledge history of dependence, and allow person and professional to discuss fears of re-activation of dependency.

➤ Explain any intent to use opioids or other psychoactive medications.

➤ Respect person's right to decide whether or not to be administered opioids.

Education of the individual

➤ Explain health risks associated with unrelieved pain, including risk of relapse.

➤ Explain that the known risk for re-activation of dependency to opioids in the context of pain is small.

➤ Ensure the person understands differences between psychological and physical dependence.

Minimise withdrawal following procedure or treatment

➤ Taper opioid analgesics *slowly* to minimise emergence of withdrawal symptoms.

➤ Assess for presence of withdrawal symptoms at least p.i.d. during analgesic taper; treat symptomatically.

➤ Offer non-pharmacological and non-opioid analgesic alternatives.

Support abstinence

➤ Encourage the person to increase contact with family and/or significant other supports. Reassure the person that it is acceptable to take medications for medical reasons. Offer to advise/reassure significant others if required.

➤ Request consultation from substance use medicine specialist.

➤ Request consultation from allied health professionals to devise pain management plans to support and minimise analgesic requirements.

➤ Screen for mental health and substance use conditions. Arrange diagnosis and treatment including referral if necessary.

➤ Include family in plan of pain care.

➤ If relapse occurs, intensify abstinence efforts; *do not terminate pain care.*[53]

Individuals on naltrexone for alcohol or opioid dependence

➤ Cease naltrexone prior to pain-producing procedures if possible. Encourage the person to seek additional support as required to maintain abstinence during this period (3–5 days), and caution opioid-dependent individuals about the risk of inadvertent overdose with relapse.

➤ In the initial 24-hour period as the naltrexone begins to wear off, the following multimodal analgesic regimes are recommended:
  — non-steroidal anti-inflammatories (e.g. ibuprofen)
  — paracetamol
  — ketamine
  — tramadol
  — regional nerve blocks/anaesthetics.

➤ *Caution.* There is experimental evidence of opioid receptor upregulation following naltrexone/opioid antagonist withdrawal. Therefore abrupt discontinuation of naltrexone may lead to increased opioid sensitivity and possibility of opioid toxicity/overdose with opioid administration. Increased supervision and monitoring is encouraged during this time. Dose administration in smaller increments may be warranted to allow increased surveillance.

➤ Continued administration of naltrexone will prevent the analgesic effects of regularly used doses of codeine or opioid-based analgesia.

➤ If unable to decrease naltrexone (e.g. due to emergency department admission or for an emergency surgical procedure), the following multimodal analgesic regimes are recommended:
  — non-steroidal anti-inflammatories (e.g. ibuprofen)
  — paracetamol
  — ketamine
  — tramadol
  — regional nerve blocks/anaesthetics.

➤ If pain is not managed, the individual should be transferred to a High Dependency Unit and opioids titrated. At very high doses and in combination with opioid adjuvants:
  — non-steroidal anti-inflammatories (e.g. ibuprofen)

— paracetamol
— ketamine
— tramadol
— regional nerve blocks/anaesthetics
➤ opioids will override antagonist effects of naltrexone and provide relief. The therapeutic window may be narrow, necessitating careful monitoring for precipitous respiratory and CNS depression.[53]

Individuals experiencing chronic pain and dependence
➤ Complicated by the need to take opioids on a regular basis for the treatment of pain.
➤ Complicated by the lack of clear pathology underlying the pain experience.
➤ Complicated in that complete analgesia is not the practical goal of opioid treatment.

Treatment
➤ Address dependency issues.
➤ Use specific treatment contracts that should detail frequency of review, dispensing agreements and any specific monitoring.
➤ Define and manage physical and emotional components of pain. A range of interventions including counselling may be helpful. These might be particularly important if the painful condition has caused significant life changes or loss of function, resulting in grief and loss issues.
➤ Identify and treat mental health–substance use conditions as indicated.
➤ Person-centred care including the use of physiotherapy and occupational therapy as required, addressing pain management and functional capacity. Interventions may include:
— acupuncture
— exercise plans
— anxiety management
— mindfulness training.

Assess, monitor and document
➤ Assess, monitor and document:
— pain severity and quality
— level of function
— presence of adverse events
— opioid analgesic use
— evidence of opioid misuse
— evaluation and plan
— progress towards therapeutic goals.[59]

Therapeutic goals
➤ Includes the functional restoration of:
— physical capabilities

- psychological intactness
- family and social interactions
- degree of healthcare utilisation
- drug use for symptom control.[53]

Preparing for discharge

➤ If the individual has become dependent or remains dependent, minimise withdrawal.
➤ If already physically dependent on opioids, initiate onto long-acting, substitution medications to prevent withdrawal.
➤ If detoxification prior to discharge is agreed upon, taper opioids *slowly* to minimise the emergence of withdrawal symptoms.
➤ Monitor for emergence of withdrawal symptoms at least q.i.d., and treat aggressively and symptomatically.
➤ If discharged on opioid analgesics with limited maintenance:
  - choose a single, long-acting formulation with lower street value (e.g. methadone or long-acting morphine)
  - write prescriptions for decreasing quantities of opioids for short periods of time with no repeats. Specify frequent dispensing. Clearly communicate discharge plans and medications to all community professionals
  - specify dosing times (*not* as required)
  - assess person's level of motivation for drug treatment and encourage entry into treatment.[53]

CONCLUSION

Collaborative practice and regular consultation among the interdisciplinary team – including the specialist palliative care and mental health teams – is important to achieve a common approach and optimise treatment outcome. Involving the interdisciplinary team throughout will ensure a consistent approach to the identified problems, improve understanding of the nature of the pain and facilitate communication.

The key to effective pain management is continuous assessment and restructuring of interventions as directed by the individual or family. The individual and family are the experts in appreciating the complexity of the pain and the best way to treat it.

The role of the family is pivotal. They should never be excluded from pain assessment. It is difficult to overstate how extremely distressing it is to see one's partner, sibling or child in chronic, unrelieved pain. Therefore:

➤ inclusion
➤ support
➤ guidance
➤ intervention
➤ opportunity to discuss how the individual feels

are imperative if therapeutic intervention is to be successful.

KEY POINT 8.18

It is important to continue supporting the individual even when interventions have not proved successful. Being present and *alongside* is a therapeutic intervention, encourages the therapeutic relationship and can be powerfully healing.

Taking care of the individual and family is pivotal. However, of equal importance is that professionals need to take care of themselves. Being with someone in pain and deep distress is emotionally draining. Discussing ones feelings about the situation and seeking support, within the context of regular supervision and good management, is not a failing. It is good quality practice and is essential if our interventions on behalf of the individual and family are to be effective.

Dependency, for people receiving opioids for dependency treatment or chronic pain, produces changes on a neurophysiological, psychological and societal level. In particular, there are the neural changes of opioid tolerance and hyperalgesia. Physical dependence and tolerance are predictable consequences of frequent opioid exposure, and alone do not indicate maladaptive behaviour.

KEY POINT 8.19

As a result of tolerance, people maintained on opioids will receive less analgesia from a given dose than people who are opioid naïve. Tolerant people will require higher opioid doses to manage acute severe pain.

KEY POINT 8.20

Maintenance opioids do not provide pain relief.

Iatrogenic dependency and relapse of dependency may occur as a result of effective management of acute severe pain, but are more likely to occur with suboptimal management of pain. Suboptimal management of pain is also likely to produce a variety of pseudo-dependent behaviours in a person's effort to ensure adequate pain relief.

Good practice should demonstrate a sound understanding of the pharmacodynamics and pharmacokinetics of pain medication in the context of opioid maintenance to prescribe, monitor and assess pain in this population effectively.

KEY POINT 8.21

It is important that professionals do not allow concerns of being manipulated to cloud their judgement concerning the individual's pain experience and lead them to providing suboptimal acute severe pain management.

Careful monitoring and aggressive pain management will reassure the person, facilitate both physical and psychological recovery, and ensure the most effective management of both pain and dependency issues.

REFERENCES

1 Chou R, Fanciullo GJ, Fine PG, *et al.* Clinical guidelines for the use of chronic opioid therapy in chronic noncancer pain. *Journal of Pain.* 2009; **10**: 113–30.

2 Alford DP, Compton P, Samet JH. Acute pain management for patients receiving maintenance methadone or buprenorphine therapy. *Annals of Internal Medicine.* 2006; **144**: 127–34.

3 Twycross R. *Introducing Palliative Care.* 4th ed. Oxford: Radcliffe Medical Press; 1999.

4 Dudgeon D, Raubertas R, Rosenthal S. The short-form McGill pain questionnaire in chronic cancer pain. *Journal of Pain and Symptoms Management.* 1993; **8**: 191–5.

5 Murdoch J, Larsen D. Assessing pain in cognitively impaired older adults. *Nursing Standard.* 2004; **18**: 33–9.

6 Abbey J, Piller N, Debellis A, *et al.* The Abbey pain scale: a 1-minute numerical indicator for people with end-stage dementia. *International Journal of Palliative Nursing.* 2004; **10**: 6–13.

7 Doloplus. *Why Doloplus?* Available at: www.doloplus.com/pourquoi/pourquoi.php (accessed 9 March 2014).

8 Hanks G, Cherney N, Christakis N, *et al.*, editors. *Oxford Textbook of Palliative Medicine.* 4th ed. Oxford: Oxford University Press; 2011. p. 600.

9 Chandler A, Preece J, Lister S. Using heat therapy for pain management. *Nursing Standard.* 2002; **17**: 40–2.

10 World Health Organization. *Cancer Pain Relief.* 2nd ed. Geneva: World Health Organization; 1996.

11 Twycross R, Wilcock A, Charlesworth S, *et al. Palliative Care Formulary.* 2nd ed. Oxford: Radcliffe Medical Press; 2002. p. 174.

12 Hanks G, Hoskin P, Aherne G, *et al.* Explanation for potency of repeated oral doses of morphine? *Lancet.* 1987; **2**(8561): 723–5.

13 Davis M, Walsh D. Rapid opioid titration in severe cancer pain. *European Journal of Palliative Care.* 2005; **12**: 11–14.

14 Hanks G, de Conno F, Cherney N, *et al.* Morphine and alternative opioids in cancer pain: the EAPC recommendations. *British Journal of Cancer.* 2001; **85**: 587–93.

15 Vadalouca A, Moka E, Argyra E, *et al.* Opioid rotation for cancer patients: a review of the literature. *Journal of Opioid Management.* 2008; **4**: 213–50.

16 Kaiko R, Wallenstein M, Rogers R, *et al.* Analgesic and mood effects of heroin and morphine in cancer patients with post-operative pain. *The New England Journal of Medicine.* 1981; **304**: 1501–5.

17 Twycross R, Wilcock A, Charlesworth S, *et al. Palliative Care Formulary.* 2nd ed. Oxford: Radcliffe Medical Press; 2002. pp. 186–7.

18 Ahmedzai S, Brooks D. Trans-dermal fentanyl versus sustained-release oral morphine in cancer pain: preference, efficacy, and quality of life. The TTS-fentanyl – comparative trial group. *Journal of Pain and Symptom Management.* 1997; **13**: 254–61.

19 Ellershaw J, Kinder C, Aldridge J, *et al.* Care of the dying: is pain control compromised or enhanced by continuation of the fentanyl trans-dermal patch in the dying phase? *Journal of Pain and Symptom Management.* 2002; **24**: 398–403.

20 Back I. *Pain in Palliative Medicine Handbook.* 3rd ed. Cardiff: BPM Books; 2001. p. 77.

21 Gibbs M. The role of transdermal fentanyl patches in the effective management of cancer pain. *International Journal of Palliative Nursing.* 2009; **15**: 354–9.

22 Twycross R, Wilcock A. *Symptom Management in Advanced Cancer*. 3rd ed. Oxford: Radcliffe Medical Press; 2001. p. 381.

23 Hanks G, Nugent M, Higgs C, *et al*. Oral transmucosal fentanyl citrate in the management of breakthrough pain in cancer: an open, multicentre, dose-titration and long-term use study. *Palliative Medicine*. 2004; **18**: 698–704.

24 Flock P, Gibbs L, Sykes N. Diamorphine-metronidazole gel effective for treatment of painful infected leg ulcers. *Journal of Pain and Symptom Management*. 2000; **20**: 396–7.

25 Grocott P. Palliative management of fungating malignant wounds. *Journal of Community Nursing*. 2000; **14**: 31–40.

26 Naylor W. Assessment and management of pain in fungating wounds. *British Journal of Nursing*. 2001; Suppl. **10**: 33–56.

27 Zepetella G. Topical opioids for painful skin ulcers: do they work? *European Journal of Palliative Care*. 2004 **11**: 93–6.

28 Naylor W. Malignant wounds: aetiology and principles of management. *Nursing Standard*. 2002; **16**: 45–53.

29 Doyle D, Hanks G, Cherny N. *Oxford Textbook of Palliative Care*. 3rd ed. Oxford: Oxford University Press; 2003.

30 Mercadante S, Villari P, Ferrera P, *et al*. Addition of a second opioid responses in cancer pain: preliminary data. *Support Cancer Care*. 2004; **12**: 762–6.

31 Toscani F, Piva L, Corli O, *et al*. Ketorolac versus diclofenac sodium in cancer pain. *Arzneimittel Forschung – Drug Research*. 1994; **44**: 550–4.

32 Buckley M, Brogden R. Ketorolac: a review of its pharmacodynamic and pharmacokinetic properties and therapeutic potential. *Drugs*. 1990; **39**: 86–109.

33 Blackwell N, Bangham L, Hughes M, *et al*. Subcutaneous keterolac – a new development in pain control. *Palliative Medicine*. 1993; **7**: 63–5.

34 Micaela M, Brogen B, Brogen R. Keterolac – a review of its pharmacodynamic and pharmacokinetic properties, and therapeutic potential. *Drugs*. 1990; **39**: 86–109.

35 Regnard C, Dean M. *A Guide to Symptom Relief in Palliative Care*. 6th ed. Oxford: Radcliffe Publishing; 2010. p. 70.

36 Johnson A. Use of bisphosphonates for the treatment of metastatic bone pain; a survey of palliative care physicians in the UK. *Palliative Medicine*. 2001; **15**: 141–7.

37 Ripamonti C, Fulfaro F, Ticozzi C, *et al*. Role of pamidronate disodium in the treatment of metastatic bone disease. *Tumori*. 1998; **84**: 442–55.

38 Body J, Deal I, Bell R, *et al*. Oral ibandronate improves bone pain and preserves quality of life in patients with skeletal metastases due to breast cancer. *Pain*. 2004; **111**: 306–12.

39 Twycross R, Wilcock A. *Pain Relief in Symptom Management in Advanced Cancer*. 3rd ed. Oxford: Radcliffe Medical Press; 2001. p. 27.

40 Osterland H, Beirne P. Complementary therapies. In: Ferrell B, Coyle N, editors. *Textbook of Palliative Nursing*. Oxford: Oxford University Press; 2001. pp. 374–5.

41 Nilsson S, Strang P, Ginman C, *et al*. Palliation of bone pain in prostate cancer using chemotherapy and Strontium-89 – a randomized phase II study. *Journal of Pain and Symptom Management*. 2005; **29**: 352–7.

42 Kaye P. *A–Z Pocketbook of Symptom Control*. Northampton: EPL Publications; 2003. p. 112.

43 Eisenberg E, River Y, Shifrin A, *et al*. Antiepileptic drugs in the treatment of neuropathic pain. *Drugs*. 2007; **67**: 1265–89.

44 Freynhagen R, Strojek K, Greising T, *et al*. Efficacy of Pregabalin in neuropathic pain evaluated in a 12-week, randomised, double-blind, multicentre, placebo-controlled trial of flexible- and fixed-dose regimens. *Pain*. 2005; **115**: 254–63.

45 Twycross R, Wilcock A, editors. *Palliative Care Formulary*. 4th ed. Nottingham: palliativedrugs.com; 2011. p. 491.

46 Edwards A, Gerrard G. The management of cerebral metastases. *European Journal of Palliative Care*. 1998; **5**: 7–11.

47 Poole D. Use of TENS in pain management, part 2: how to use TENS. *Nursing Times*. 2007; **103**: 28–9.

48 Saunders C. *Hospice and Palliative Care: an interdisciplinary approach*. London: Edward Arnold; 1990. p. 27.

49 Stimmel B. *Pain and its Relief Without Addiction*. New York: Haworth Medical Press; 1997. p. 77.

50 Coyle N, Ferrel B, editors. *Oxford Textbook of Palliative Nursing*. 3rd ed. New York, NY: Open University Press; 2010. p. 172.

51 McCaffrey M, Pasero C. *Pain: clinical manual*. 2nd ed. London: Mosby; 1999.

52 Athanasos P, Smith CS, White JM, *et al*. Methadone maintenance patients are cross-tolerant to the antinociceptive effects of very high plasma morphine concentrations. *Pain*. 2006; **120**: 267–75.

53 Compton P, Athanasos P, de Crespigny C. *Opioid Tolerance and the Effective Management of Acute Pain*. Sydney: Drug and Alcohol Nurses of Australasia Conference; 2006.

54 Rapp SE, Ready LB, Nessly ML. Acute pain management in patients with prior opioid consumption: a case-controlled retrospective review. *The Journal of Pain*. 1995; **61**: 195–201.

55 de Leon-Casasola OA, Myers DP, Donaparthi S, *et al*. A comparison of postoperative epidural analgesia between patients with chronic cancer taking high doses of oral opioids versus opioid-naive patients. *Anesthesia and Analgesia*. 1993; **76**: 302–7.

56 Hay JL, White JM, Bochner F, *et al*. Hyperalgesia in opioid-managed chronic pain and opioid-dependent patients. *Journal of Pain*. 2009; **3**: 316–22.

57 Schnoll SH, Weaver MF. Addiction and pain. *American Journal of Addiction*. 2003; **12**(Suppl. 2): S27–35.

58 Parish JM. Sleep-related problems in common medical conditions. *Chest*. 2009; **135**: 563–72.

59 Passik SD, Kirsh KL. The need to identify predictors of aberrant drug-related behavior and addiction in patients being treated with opioids for pain. *Pain Medicine*. 2003; **4**: 186–9.

TO LEARN MORE

- Basford L. Complementary therapies. In: Basford L, Slevin O, editors. *Theory and Practice of Nursing: an integrated approach to caring*. 2nd ed. Cheltenham: Nelson Thornes; 2003. pp. 569–96.
- Behavioural pain assessment scale and discussion for older patients with verbal communication disorders. Available at: www.doloplus.com/pourquoi/pourquoi.php (accessed 9 March 2014).
- British Pain Society. Available at: www.britishpainsociety.org/index.html (accessed 9 March 2014).
- Cooper J, editor. *Stepping into Palliative Care 1: relationships and responses*. Oxford: Radcliffe Medical Press; 2006.
- Cooper J, editor. *Stepping into Palliative Care 2: care and practice*. Oxford: Radcliffe Medical Press; 2006.
- Discussion of pharmaceutical and other treatment of pain. Available at: www.palliativedrugs.com/index.html (accessed 9 March 2014).
- Hanks G, Cherny NI, Christakis NA, *et al*. editors. *Oxford Textbook of Palliative Medicine*. 4th ed. Oxford: Oxford University Press; 2011.
- Information on TENS machine settings. Available at: www.electrotherapy.org (accessed 23 April 2012).
- International Association for Pain and Chemical Dependency. Available at: www.iapcd.org (accessed 9 March 2014).
- Regnard C, Dean M. *A Guide to Symptom Relief in Advanced Disease*. 6th ed. Oxford: Radcliffe Publishing; 2010.
- Relaxation exercises. Available at: www.patient.co.uk/showdoc/27000363/ (accessed 9 March 2014).

- Smith H, Passik S. *Pain and Chemical Dependency*. New York, NY: Oxford University Press; 2008.
- Stimmel B. *Pain and its Relief without Addiction: clinical issues in the use of opioids and other analgesics*. Birmingham, NY: Haworth Medical Press; 1997.
- Twycross R, Wilcock A, Stark Toller C. *Symptom Management in Advanced Cancer*. 4th ed. Nottingham: palliativedrugs.com; 2009.
- Twycross R, Wilcock A, editors. *Palliative Care Formulary*. 4th ed. Nottingham: palliativedrugs.com; 2011.
- Wall P. *Pain: the Science of Suffering*. New York, NY: Columbia University Press; 2002.

ACKNOWLEDGEMENT

The authors are grateful to the editors and publishers for permitting adaptation of the following chapters: Mitten T. Introduction to pain management. In: Cooper J, editor. *Stepping into Palliative Care 2: care and practice*. 2nd ed. Oxford: Radcliffe Publishing; 2006. pp. 16–39; Athanasos P, Neild R, de Crespigny C, *et al*. Pain management. In Cooper DB, editor. *Care in Mental Health–Substance Use*. London: Radcliffe Publishing; 2011. pp. 215–28.

ANSWER TO SELF-ASSESSMENT EXERCISE 8.4 (*SEE* P. 117)

Lisa might have become agitated from having uncontrolled pain due to her fracture. Her pain may be uncontrolled due to lack of analgesia or inadequate analgesia. Lisa may also be experiencing emerging withdrawal syndrome from one or both of her drugs of dependence. Information from Lisa's methadone treatment provider is necessary. This will confirm her current dose and dosing schedule, including information to confirm the last dose given and any take-away doses. Information about observed dosing will help to establish the likelihood of diversion of Lisa's prescribed methadone.

Confirmation of the results of Lisa's most recent urine drug screen will also be useful. It is important to confirm the type of urine drug screen test that was performed when Lisa was admitted to hospital as not all standard screens will detect methadone. The hospital laboratory will provide this information. Any recent medication changes are important to be aware of as some medications may significantly alter the metabolism of methadone. A serum methadone level (blood test) may be useful in cases such as this.

After confirming Lisa's methadone treatment dose and establishing confidence that she is currently taking her methadone, her regular dose should be given. This regular dose will not provide any analgesia for her acute pain. Intra-operative pain relief should be given as usual and short-acting opioids should be titrated to effect. Post-operatively, long-acting opioids should be given with short-acting agents titrated for breakthrough pain. Non-opioid pain relief should also be used and may remain as part of the treatment plan as opioid analgesia is reduced after the initial effects of the injury begin to settle.

Lisa may have been receiving take-away doses of methadone and diverting these doses elsewhere. This would have resulted in a negative urine screen for methadone. If there is any doubt as to Lisa's compliance with her current methadone treatment (concern about potential diversion), the overall dose may be reduced and given as a split dose. Short-acting analgesic agents should be titrated to effect. Consultation with her usual methadone treatment providers should be sought in this instance to promote restabilisation prior to discharge.

Lisa should be reassured that her pain will be treated. She should be told that it could sometimes be somewhat more complicated to treat pain in those on methadone maintenance treatment but that staff will not give up until her pain is adequately treated. An explanation of the relevance of her recent drug use history including the illicit use of drugs and pharmaceuticals should be given alongside reassurance that any information given will be used solely to optimise her treatment.

CHAPTER 9

The young person and suicide

Philip James

INTRODUCTION

Suicide is an emotive issue and it could be argued that because the act of suicide results in death, it is one of the most important and challenging issues for mental health professionals. Once a person has died there are no second chances to address the problem, and this pressure contributes to some dramatic and understandable responses. It is important to bear in mind that suicidality is a symptom that often accompanies emotional problems, but it is important that when dealing with suicidality the underlying problems do not get ignored.

In addition to clarifying and explaining the various jargon associated with self-harm and suicidality, this chapter argues that many of the modern approaches to dealing with suicidality frequently do lose sight of the problem behind the suicidality. It will be suggested that many of the features of palliative care, such as the focus on person-centredness, respect of autonomy and an openness to discuss quality of life issues, should be at the heart of working with those who are suicidal. It will be further suggested that the principles of motivational interviewing, an approach developed to help resolve ambivalence among those misusing substances, is ideal for working with people who are thinking of ending their own life.

UNDERSTANDING THE JARGON

Like most areas of healthcare, and possibly as a measure of the importance with which this area is regarded, a lot has been written on this topic. Consequently, various terms have come into use over the decades and it is important to outline them carefully.

Self-destructive behaviours

Self-destructive behaviours is a very broad term used to describe a situation where an individual engages in behaviours that are harmful to them. These behaviours could vary from behaviours where the intention is not necessarily to harm oneself, such as smoking cigarettes or nail biting, to behaviours such as deliberately cutting or burning him- or herself. The harm does not have to be physical and could even include social or emotional harms. Completed suicide can also be included as a self-destructive behaviour.[1]

Deliberate self-harm

Deliberate self-harm (DSH) is a term commonly used to describe deliberate acts that the person engages in, knowing that this will cause harm to her- or himself. The behaviours can vary from cutting, burning, scratching and biting. Some authors include behaviours such as tattooing and piercing. This makes examining rates a little difficult as the definition used in any study can change the rates considerably. That being said, rates of DSH can be quite high and can vary significantly from country to country and by gender. A large study of over 30,000 15–16 year olds from seven countries reported lifetime rates of 4.3% for males and 13.5% for females.[2] However, the rates varied drastically, with 17% of Australian girls having self-harmed compared to only 5.7% in the Netherlands.

Suicidal ideation

Suicidal ideation (SI) is a term often used to describe a situation where the individual is thinking about suicide. It is important to remember that the intensity and frequency of such thoughts can vary considerably, from the person intermittently thinking 'I would be better off dead' to a pervasive thought that he or she should kill her- or himself. A large general population study of over 12,000 adults in five European countries examined the rates of suicidal ideation or thoughts and found that 9.5% of respondents had experienced some suicidal ideation in the previous two weeks.[3] Among those who had some form of suicidal thought, less than 1 in 10 (or 1% of the general population) indicated that they would like to kill themselves or would kill themselves if they had a chance. The others indicated that they simply have thoughts of killing themselves.

Suicide attempt

Suicide attempt is relatively easy to define – it is simply when someone makes some form of deliberate effort to take their own life, which may or may not be successful. The main difference here is that the intention is for the person to kill themselves, which is not always the case in DSH. However, it can be difficult in practice to conclusively say whether an individual incident is a suicide attempt. Many professionals working in mental health services will have met people who clearly state they were trying to kill themselves following an episode of self-harm. But based upon the methods they used or the timing of the attempt, the professional may have their doubts. For example, an individual may take an overdose of the exact same dose of a medication which previously had not proved fatal, raising questions about their determination to kill themselves.

Completed suicide

Completed suicide is when the individual's attempt to kill him- or herself is successful. According to the World Health Organization (WHO) the international suicide rate is 16 people per 100,000 population.[4] There is considerable variance between countries and according to age and gender, with young men at particularly high risk of killing themselves.

Parasuicide

Parasuicide is a term that seems to have fallen out of use in recent years but was used as an umbrella term to include DSH and suicide attempt. In general it is used to describe a self-inflicted act that looks like suicide without actually being fatal – although some writers have included completed suicide within their definition of parasuicide.

What these terms and figures show us is that suicidality exists on a continuum, ranging from a person having vague thoughts that she or he would be better off dead, to plans to actually kill her- or himself. This is represented in Figure 9.1. While graphically this appears like a one-way system with clearly defined stages, this is not the case in reality. Level of suicidality can vary over time and often over a relatively short period of time, such as hours.

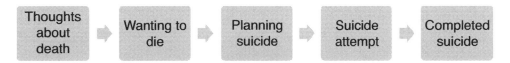

Figure 9.1

It is worth highlighting that while thoughts about suicide are relatively common (9.5% of people in the past 2 weeks)[3] only 0.016% of people per year actually complete suicide according to the WHO statistics. This makes assessing and preventing suicide notoriously difficult for professionals for the simple reason that even among those who are expressing suicidal thoughts, and there are a lot in this group, relatively few will actually complete suicide.

REFLECTIVE PRACTICE EXERCISE 9.1

> **Time: 20 minutes**
> Think about some of the people who have engaged in deliberate self-harm (DSH), or thought about DSH, whom you have encountered in the course of your work. Ask yourself the following questions:
> * What did these people hope to achieve by their behaviour?
> * Were they all trying to kill themselves?
> * Was it always easy to identify how serious the suicide risk was?
> * Did the suicide risk remain stable throughout the course of a day or week?
> * What interventions did you make to reduce the risk of suicide?

KEY POINT 9.1

Suicidality exists on a continuum with about 9.5% of people thinking about suicide per fortnight but relatively few people actually completing suicide. This makes it difficult to identify those most at risk.

WHY DO PEOPLE WANT TO KILL THEMSELVES?

This is a very difficult question that has plagued mental health researchers for decades and it is certain that no conclusive answer has been found. History is littered with examples of people taking their own lives for a variety of reasons. The photo of the Buddhist Monk Thich Quang Duc setting himself on fire in Saigon in protest against the Vietnamese government is one of the most famous images of the 1960s (see http:// en.wikipedia.org/wiki/Thich_Quang_Duc – accessed 11 March 2014). However, it may not be commonly associated with suicide. There is no simple reason why people decide to kill themselves and Box 9.1 provides some explanations for why people might want to kill themselves.

BOX 9.1 Why people want to kill themselves

Brain or biological disorder
There is a growing body of literature that suggests that those who are suicidal often have differences in their brain. This can be linked with hopelessness, an inability to think of other options and depression.[5]

Life situations
Many people become suicidal in response to extreme life events such as job loss or relationship breakdown.

Poor coping ability
Those who are suicidal may have poor or impaired ability to cope or deal with stressors and consequently are more prone to becoming suicidal.

Social acceptability
Suicide is more common in certain societies. It can be argued that changes in society can make suicide appear like a more realistic solution to some people. This can explain the phenomenon of clusters of suicides where one suicide can lead to a spike in suicides in that area.

Drugs and alcohol
There is no doubt that alcohol and drugs impair an individual's ability to deal with problems. A study in Ireland found that 11 out of 12 people under 30 years old who killed themselves had taken alcohol at the time.[6]

Political/altruistic motive
Where a person gives her or his life to save another individual or to highlight the plight of others. Thich Quang Duc's self-immolation described above could be seen as an example, as could the idea of suicide bombers or kamikaze pilots (World War II).

Avoiding something
In many cases it appears that people choose suicide as it appears to be a way of avoiding something negative. Euthanasia could be a way of avoiding a painful death (*see* Chapter 13).

Examining the descriptions of suicide given above we can clearly see that there is a huge amount of overlap between them. For example, a young man who chooses to kill himself in response to the break-up of a relationship may see himself as belonging to the final category – he is simply avoiding the awful situation of living without his girlfriend. However, the professionals that come in contact with him may have a considerably different view of this and may actually believe he has a brain disorder such as depression or a poor ability at coping that could be seen as a psychological problem. Another professional may put it down to his unhealthy use of alcohol. The view taken as to the cause of suicidality has a significant influence on the way services deal with suicidal individuals.

KEY POINT 9.2

People's reasons for wanting to take their own life are varied and complicated. Simply attributing suicide to the person being depressed is an oversimplification.

MENTAL HEALTH RESPONSE TO SUICIDE

It is important to stress that facilities and services available for people vary from country to country and not all health services are the same. However, as a general rule mental health services are the main port of call for those who present with significant thoughts of suicide. As suicide is a leading cause of death among young people, there is a growing body of work and literature based around suicide prevention. For example, in September 2013 there was a National Suicide Prevention Week (UK), with lots of effort going into making people more aware of suicide risk and trying to help those who are suicidal.

Those who are suicidal are generally referred to the mental health services and seen by a psychiatrist. This assessment is aimed at identifying the level of suicide risk and putting in place appropriate treatment plans for people. In cases where the risk of suicide is high this may include admission to a mental health inpatient unit or referral to a community mental health team. When the risk is deemed to be lower (and there is no evidence of a mental health problem such as depression) the person may be referred to a community service outside of the mental health service such as a counselling service.

This might appear relatively straightforward, but in reality the picture is quite different. In cases where alcohol or other substances are seen to play a significant role in the person's difficulties they are often referred to the substance use (which includes alcohol and other drugs) service and not offered 'mental health' care. Alternatively, the assessment may lead to a decision that as no mental health diagnosis, particularly depression, is apparent, the person is not deemed to be appropriate for the mental health services and so no treatment is offered. Such decisions often lead to hurt and confusion for the suicidal person and their family, who feel under immense pressure to protect their loved one. This hurt is probably amplified because suicide prevention campaigns are often encouraging loved ones to be vigilant for those who are at risk of suicide. Not being offered a service once their suicidal loved one is brought to the service's attention appears nonsensical to relatives. Case Study 9.1 illustrates this point.

Case Study 9.1

Mike (23) lives with his parents. Recently he has been feeling down following the break-up of a relationship with his girlfriend. He has become increasingly withdrawn and his parents have become worried about him. His parents arrive home on a Friday night to find him sitting in the dark in the kitchen with a length of rope on his lap. Mike is tearful and says he just could not bring himself to go through with his plan to hang himself.

His parents phone the emergency services and as it is outside of office hours an ambulance brings Mike to the local accident and emergency department. He is triaged and referred to the on-call psychiatrist. The psychiatrist met with him for about an hour and asked Mike all about his thoughts of suicide. The psychiatrist told Mike that he did not have depression or any other mental illness. He further said that he thinks Mike's suicidal thoughts were related to his alcohol intake (Mike admitted to drinking about seven pints of lager earlier in the evening) and said he would refer him to the local substance use services for counselling. Mike was deemed to be no longer at risk and was sent home with his parents after seven hours in the accident and emergency department. He feels the doctor totally dismissed his upset about his girlfriend once he was aware of his alcohol intake. Mike does not think he has a drink problem and has no intention of going to see an alcohol counsellor. His parents are very upset and cannot understand how Mike could not be offered a service given how suicidal he was.

SELF-ASSESSMENT EXERCISE 9.1

Time: 10 minutes
Given the palliative care principles and philosophy, how might this situation be managed in a more positive and compassionate way?

Although Mike was offered referral to an alcohol service, he and his parents do not see this as appropriate as he was looking for help with his mood. Given how distressed he was, it seems incomprehensible to both Mike and his family that the mental health service have not offered him further appointments.

REFLECTIVE PRACTICE EXERCISE 9.2

Time: 10 minutes
Reflect on how this might impact on the feelings of Mike's family.

However, for those who are admitted into mental health units, care is often experienced as less than adequate. Naturally, when people are admitted into mental health units the primary focus is on maintaining their safety and so the unit environment is designed to reduce the opportunities to cause harm to oneself. Items that can be used to cut oneself may be replaced with less harmful alternatives – for example unbreakable glass. Observation, where a nurse keeps the individual in view at all times, restricting leave from the unit, may also be used. Professionals then have to strike a balance between excessive restrictions, which may increase a person's wish to die, and keeping him or her safe.[7] Such observation methods led one hospitalised individual to comment that they were forced into the role of 'early feminists' as they would not shave their legs because to do so would require them to have a nurse in the bathroom with them.[8] Another common method used by mental health professionals is for the individual to sign a suicide contract, which is an agreement that the person will not harm him- or herself and will speak to a member of the team if he or she feels like doing so. However, there is little evidence of their effectiveness, leading many to caution against reliance on them in practice.[9,10]

The current mental health approach has received a further blow following the publication of a large study examining the effect of the introduction of new mental health policies and legislation in 100 countries. Perhaps surprisingly, this study found that the introduction of mental health policies or legislation in a country actually *increased* the rates of suicide in that country.[11] In fact, this study found that only the introduction of substance use policies was actually associated with a reduction in suicide, raising considerable questions about how we approach those in mental health distress. Research seems to indicate that for many individuals, the things they find most useful about mental health services is the opportunity to talk to a professional about their problems.[12] This has led to a more person-centred approach, such as the Tidal Model, where affording people an opportunity to talk about their situation is the focus.[13]

KEY POINT 9.3

When individuals who feel suicidal approach mental health services they do not always experience it as useful. They often believe that the focus of attention is not where they feel it ought to be.

THE PRINCIPLES OF PALLIATIVE CARE

Recently it has been purported that the principles underlying palliative care could provide a useful guide to providing this more person-centred approach to care.[14] While traditionally palliative care has been related to the provision of care to those who are dying, it has developed into a standalone theory or philosophy of caring. Cooper and Cooper[14] outline various principles and philosophies of palliative care that apply to mental health care including:

➤ person-centred practice

➤ relationship-based connectedness – between professional, individual and family
➤ a focus on compassion
➤ respect for autonomy and choice
➤ openness to quality of life issues
➤ the family as the unit of care.

It is clear from reading these principles that most people engaging with mental health services would see them as being an improvement. For example, most professionals believe in the idea of person-centred care, where the person is treated as an individual with a specific care plan formulated between him or her and a key worker, targeting the individual's concerns. This naturally leads into the need to give due regard to the relationship between the professional and the person. This may be more difficult for services to adapt to. For example, many individuals bemoan the current system where new junior doctors seem to appear every time they attend the clinic, or key nurses are moved from unit to unit to shore up understaffed areas. However, most professionals would most likely agree that the relationship between them and the individual is important.

KEY POINT 9.4

The issue of compassion is close to the heart of so many professionals and professions.

The Oxford Dictionary defines compassion as 'sympathetic pity and concern for the sufferings or misfortunes of others',[15] and for most health professionals this is at the core of why they do their job (*see* Chapter 2).

However, this author believes that the last three philosophies will seem more challenging for many professionals to embrace. Whilst respect for autonomy and choice are easily articulated and lofty goals, are they as readily adhered to in practice? Is it even possible to adhere to them in practice? As outlined by the experience of Kaysen in the 1960s,[8] a considerable amount of energy is put into 'keeping the patient alive' by health services. Many people are detained in mental health units and treated against their will, and suicide risk is one of the major reasons for using such a coercive approach. Most professionals detest this aspect of their work and simply do it as a necessary means to keep the person alive. However, if we are allowed to detain people for treatment of their mental health problem this raises questions about the actual level of autonomy allowed to those attending the mental health services.

This also leads to a potential impasse in relation to allowing open conversations about quality of life issues. If we take Mike, who we discussed in Case Study 9.1, he raised serious questions about whether he felt his life was worth living without his girlfriend. This is a position that many people can relate to from their own experience in losing relationships. However, the conversation for people in such positions often proceeds down one of two tracks:

1 These suicidal thoughts are the symptoms of mental ill-health which requires treatment.
2 This is not a valid mental health or emotional problem as it is simply the effect or symptom of a different problem, e.g. alcohol use – as is the case for Mike.

Neither of these responses is wholly satisfactory for the same reason – neither of them acknowledge the level of upset and perspective that the person has, namely that life may not be worth living. We know from research and the figures discussed earlier that the vast majority of people who experience suicidal thoughts never go on to complete suicide, but thinking of suicide is a common human response to difficulties in life.

Maltsberger[16] eloquently articulates the difficulties that can unfold in cases where professionals are asked to work with people who present with significant self-harm or suicidality. Suicidality typically evokes strong 'counter suicide' responses in the professional they encounter.[16] As outlined earlier, the measures used may include committal to inpatient mental health care, special observations and the removal of various freedoms and items in order to ensure the person's safety. In doing so, the professional assumes an inordinate amount of responsibility to keep the individual safe from him- or herself. At first glance, such responses seem justifiable and even vital if the person is to be kept alive. However, it is hard to argue that such responses fit neatly with the palliative principle of respecting an individual's right to autonomy and choice. Moreover, it is likely that conversations regarding quality of life may also be unlikely to occur, as the person's suicidality is seen as a symptom of their mental health problem. This further impinges on a service's ability to have an open conversation on quality of life issues. Individuals who are attending mental health services may soon learn that it is not a good idea to discuss suicidal thoughts with mental health professionals.

This author contends that in many cases the current approaches to discussing (or not discussing for that matter) a person's suicidal thoughts and ideas is not only a missed opportunity to intervene but could also make the situation worse. By the application of motivational interviewing, the professional is able to engage in a more open and person-centred way with the person about her or his suicidality and actually reduce the person's suicidality.

KEY POINT 9.5

By applying the principles of palliative care to the person who is suicidal, the professional will be required to engage in a more meaningful and engaging way with the individual, thus avoiding restrictive and paternalistic practices.

MOTIVATIONAL INTERVIEWING AND SUICIDALITY

Motivational interviewing (MI) is an approach to counselling or having a conversation with someone in a bid to reduce their ambivalence and promote behaviour change. It was originally developed in the early 1980s by psychologists Bill Miller and Stephen

Rollnick as a method of working with people experiencing alcohol problems who were ambivalent about making changes. Since then it has been applied to a variety of health-related areas and more recently mental health problems.[17] In developing MI, Miller and Rollnick made a number of impressive and important breakthroughs in understanding an individual's motivation.

Understanding ambivalence

One of the key concepts of MI is the recognition that many individuals presenting to mental health and counselling services are ambivalent or undecided about changing. It is easy to see how this may apply to substance use – someone may on one hand believe that their drinking is causing them significant harm and damaging their relationships, while at the same time, believing that it helps them relax and makes it easier for them to mix with people. This ambivalence freezes the person in terms of action, as they can see both advantages and disadvantages of stopping. Miller and Rollnick named this situation 'the decisional imbalance'.[18] It is fair to say that the decisional imbalance applies equally as well to those who are suicidal. Many people who are thinking of killing themselves can see both pros and cons of doing so, and this often explains why they have not yet done so.

KEY POINT 9.6

If the person is frozen in inaction by the question of whether or not to kill her- or himself, this often means that she or he is not working on improving his or her life either, thus perpetuating the problems.

The analysis of the person's ambivalence often leads to an examination of two questions:
1 Do I want to live?
2 Do I want to die?[19]

By allowing an exploration of the pros and cons of these two questions the professional now has the opportunity to help the individual to resolve this ambivalence. As the individual and professional discuss these questions, the person often achieves a new perspective on the situation – he or she does not actually want to die but simply feels that there is little choice as he or she cannot see a way out of these current problems.[19] Table 9.1 contains an illustration of what an exploration of Mike's (Case Study 9.1) decisional imbalance might look like. Such an approach requires the professional to accept that while suicide is not a desirable outcome, it is one choice the person has. While admission to mental health care and 24-hour observation make it more difficult for the person to kill her- or himself, the person cannot guarantee that suicide will not happen. However, such an approach does not allow the person-centred discussion of the choices and a respect for the end-of-life issues advocated by palliative care.[14]

TABLE 9.1 Mike's decisional imbalance for his suicidal thoughts

Pros of living	*Cons of living*
• I might be able to be happy • My family will not have to deal with my suicide • I will be able to work on the other goals I had for my life	• I might always feel this bad
Pros of dying	*Cons of dying*
• I will not feel like I do now	• It will have a huge negative effect on my family • I will never know if I would be able to sort things out • There's no second chance

Change talk

Another important contribution to the area of healthcare made by MI is the concept of change talk. Miller and Rollnick[19] recognised that those who voiced reasons about why they would like to change or what would be better for them if they changed, were more likely to change. This finding has subsequently been validated by empirical research.[20] Miller and Rollnick coined the term 'change talk' to describe this type of speech. However, perhaps even more importantly, they discovered that statements made by a professional about why the individual should change, or the advantages for him or her if change is made, are not correlated with change. In fact it appears to be correlated with not making a change, with the person becoming even more resistant. The resulting message for those working with people in distress is that the more we can get people to articulate the reasons why a behaviour such as suicide is not in their long-term interest, the less likely they are to act on them, but the more we voice reasons to change, the less motivated the person gets.

For many professionals this may seem counterintuitive – surely we need to convince people not to kill themselves! However, if we take a moment to think about such conversations from an MI perspective, things take on a different light. For most people, a difficult decision results in a decisional imbalance whereby they can see both positive and negative effects of both choices. Just as a person with substance use problems can see the pros and cons of reducing their alcohol or drug taking, so too can the person who is contemplating suicide see the pros and cons of doing so. Should a professional take up the side of not killing him- or herself, the person often points out the flip side and argues for the benefits of taking their own life. Consequently, the person not only feels the professional does not understand his or her predicament, but is in fact voicing reasons they should kill her- or himself. This is likely to increase the person's thoughts in relation to suicide, as illustrated by the extract in Box 9.2 related to Case Study 9.1.

BOX 9.2 Excerpt of conversation between the professional and Mike

- Professional: Think of the effect your suicide would have on your parents.
- Mike: Look, I am not stupid. I know how upset they would be, but they'll cope.
- Professional: Will they?
- Mike: Maybe, but what about me? I'm miserable. I can't go on like this.
- Professional: I think that if you were not taking so much alcohol you probably would not feel as bad as you do now.
- Mike: I am not an alcoholic, stop treating me like I am. You don't understand.

How to increase change talk

To give a full overview of the MI techniques is beyond the scope of this chapter. However, there are a number of core principles and skills that can be used. Miller and Rollnick[18] list four general principles of MI which fit neatly with the principles of palliative care as applied to mental health care by Cooper and Cooper.[14]

1 **Express empathy** – Showing understanding for someone's point of view and upset is a key skill in any helping relationship, and one of the most effective ways to do this is to express this overtly. Statements such as 'it sounds like things have been very difficult for you' and 'while you're not comfortable with the idea of killing yourself, at times you struggle to come up with a better solution', shows the person that they are being understood by the professional and encourages them to explore their situation further.

2 **Develop discrepancy** – Helping the individual to see that his or her plan or actions may not fit with their own values can help the person feel uncomfortable with this choice and help resolve ambivalence. For example, a person who has a strong belief in treating their mother well might be very uncomfortable with the upset that their suicide is likely to cause her should they go through with it. The skill for professionals is allowing a person to discover this for him- or herself, as simply telling him or her 'your mum will be devastated' often elicits resistance.

3 **Roll with resistance** – Should a person voice reasons to kill her- or himself or engage in any unhealthy behaviour for that matter, the default position for many health professionals is to challenge this. These challenges tend to entrench the individual's position as the professional takes up one side of the argument for change and the individual takes up the other side. It is deeply unhelpful if the person is arguing about why they should kill him- or herself. Resistance should be taken as a sign that the current approach is not working and a new approach needs to be employed.[18]

4 **Support self-efficacy** – If a person believes that they cannot improve their situation, then they are unlikely to work at doing so. The individual becomes hopeless and so gives up. MI encourages professionals to build on a person's self-efficacy, or to increase her or his confidence in their ability to change and cope with the problems confronting him or her. Unfortunately the sometimes necessary approach of detaining people for mental health treatment does little to increase this confidence.

Asking the individual to describe how she or he has coped with this problem for the past few weeks, for example, gets the person talking about how she or he did cope, thereby increasing confidence in their abilities.

These four principles are at the heart of MI and, as we can see, they fit neatly with the principles of palliative care outlined at the beginning of the chapter. For example, working with the person and not attempting to force him or her to not choose suicide allows a conversation regarding quality of life to be opened. In turn, the use of empathy, avoiding confrontation and building self-efficacy, allows for person-centred care, compassion and a respect for autonomy. But most importantly it allows the person to discover for him- or herself that suicide is actually unlikely to be the best solution to their problems.

KEY POINT 9.7

Motivational interviewing encourages the professional to discuss the pros and cons of a course of action in an open and non-confrontational manner. By voicing reasons why suicide is an unhelpful approach the person is likely to become less motivated to use such an approach.

CONCLUSION

This chapter highlights the concerns that in many cases mental health services have adopted a very medical, risk-assessment focus to working with individuals presenting with self-harm or suicide risks. This approach often tends to alienate the person further from treatment services and, more worryingly, may even increase the person's suicidality. By incorporating the principles of palliative care, with a greater focus on compassion, understanding the individual's experience and avoiding simple risk-avoidance strategies, services can become more responsive to the individual's needs. It could further be suggested that the principles of MI can provide an excellent framework and skill set for professionals to apply these principles.

REFERENCES

1 Riley EA, Kneisl CR. Suicide and Self-Destructive Behaviour. In: Wilson H, Kneisl CR, editors. *Psychiatric Nursing.* 5th ed. Menlo Park: Addison-Wesley Nursing; 1996. pp. 585–615.
2 Madge N, Hewitt A, Hawton K, *et al.* Deliberate self-harm within an international community sample of young people: comparative findings from the Child & Adolescent Self-harm in Europe (CASE) study. *Journal of Child Psychology and Psychiatry.* 2008; **49**: 667–77.
3 Casey P, Dunn G, Kelly BD, *et al.* The prevalence of suicidal ideation in the general population: results from the Outcome of Depression International Network (ODIN) study. *Social Psychiatry and Psychiatric Epidemiology.* 2008; **43**: 299–304.
4 World Health Organization. *Suicide Prevention (SUPRE).* 2013. Available at www.who.int/mental_health/prevention/suicide/suicideprevent/en/ (accessed 11 March 2014).

5 Oquendo MA, Placidi GP, Malone KM, *et al.* Positron emission tomography of regional brain metabolic responses to a serotonergic challenge and lethality of suicide attempts in major depression. *Archives of General Psychiatry.* 2003; **60**: 14–22.

6 Bedford D, O'Farrell A, Howell F. Blood alcohol levels in persons who died from accidents and suicide. *Irish Medical Journal.* 2006; **99**: 80–3.

7 Gallop R, Stamina E. The person who is suicidal. In: Barker P, editor. *Psychiatric and Mental Health Nursing: the craft of caring.* London: Arnold; 2003. pp. 227–35.

8 Kaysen S. *Girl, Interrupted.* London: Virgo Press; 1995.

9 American Psychiatric Association. *Practice Guidelines for the Assessment and Treatment of Patients with Suicidal Behaviours.* Arlington: American Psychiatric Association; 2003.

10 McMyler C, Pryjmachuk S. Do 'no suicide' contracts work? *Journal of Psychiatric and Mental Health Nursing.* 2008; **15**: 512–22.

11 Burgess P, Pirkis J, Jolley D, *et al.* Do nations' mental health policies, programs and legislation influence their suicide rates? An ecological study of 100 countries. *Australian and New Zealand Journal of Psychiatry.* 2004; **38**: 933–9.

12 Jackson S, Stevenson C. The gift of time from a friendly professional. *Nursing Standard.* 1998; **12**: 31–3.

13 Buchanan-Barker P, Barker P. The Tidal Model. In: Cooper DB, Cooper J, editors. *Palliative Care within Mental Health: principles and philosophy.* London/New York: Radcliffe Publishing; 2012. pp. 10–21.

14 Cooper J, Cooper DB. Embracing palliative care within mental health. In: Cooper DB, Cooper J, editors. *Palliative Care within Mental Health: principles and philosophy.* London/New York: Radcliffe Publishing; 2012. pp. 1–11.

15 Pearsall J, editor. *The Concise Oxford Dictionary.* 10th ed. Oxford: Oxford University Press. 2001; p. 290.

16 Maltsberger, JT. Calculated risks in the treatment of intractably suicidal patients. *Psychiatry.* 1994; **57**: 199–212.

17 Arkowitz H, Westra HA, Miller WR, Rollnick S, editors. *Motivational Interviewing in the Treatment of Psychological Problems.* New York: The Guilford Press; 2008.

18 Miller WR, Rollnick S. *Motivational Interviewing: preparing people for change.* 2nd ed. New York: The Guilford Press; 2002. pp. 52–84.

19 Zerler H. Motivational interviewing and suicidality. In: Arkowitz H, Westra HA, Miller WR, Rollnick S, editors. *Motivational Interviewing in the Treatment of Psychological Problems.* New York: The Guilford Press; 2008. pp. 173–93.

20 Amrhein PC, Miller WR, Yahne CE, *et al.* Client commitment language during motivational interviewing predicts drug use outcome. *Journal of Consulting and Clinical Psychology.* 2003; **71**: 862–78.

TO LEARN MORE

• Cooper DB, Cooper J, editors. *Palliative Care within Mental Health: principles and philosophy.* London/New York: Radcliffe Publishing; 2012.

• Miller WR, Rollnick S. *Motivational Interviewing: preparing people for change.* 2nd ed. New York: The Guilford Press; 2002.

• Rollnick S, Miller WR, Butler CC. *Motivational Interviewing in Health Care: helping patients change behaviour.* New York: The Guilford Press; 2002.

• Zerler H. Motivational interviewing and suicidality. In: Arkowitz H, Westra HA, Miller WR, Rollnick S, editors. *Motivational Interviewing in the Treatment of Psychological Problems.* New York: The Guilford Press; 2008. pp. 173–93.

CHAPTER 10

Long-term mental health

Alyna Turner, Stephanie Oak, Brian Kelly, Amanda L Baker

INTRODUCTION

It is estimated that 12.8–36.8% of people around the world will experience a serious and enduring mental health condition during their lifetime.[1] In contrast to transient and/or mild mental health symptoms, conditions such as schizophrenia, bipolar affective disorder, personality disorders and chronic depression ('severe mental health problems' – SMHP) can potentially take a chronic and persistent course, and can be life-changing. Many people experiencing mental health problems, particularly in less-developed countries, do not receive adequate treatment and follow-up care.[2]

Uncertainty regarding the course of SMHP is the norm. While stereotypes often paint SMHP as chronic, deteriorating and associated with poor outcomes, the evidence suggests that many people will show significant improvements in symptoms and outcomes, or even improve over time. For example, for those experiencing schizophrenia, around 14% are expected to recover over 10 years, persistently demonstrating very good clinical, social and functional outcomes,[3] while even more demonstrate significant improvements in symptoms and function. As such, the need for long-term care for many people and an awareness of the potential impact of both the condition and the treatment that these individuals and their families receive must be balanced with realistic hope.

McGorry *et al.*[4] use a staged approach to describe the pattern of change in chronic mental health problems. Not all people who are at one stage necessarily progress to the next, as remission is possible at any stage. While such a model has been controversial,[5] it is an example of efforts to utilise clinical staging, particularly relevant to conditions such as schizophrenia. The earliest stage is the point of being at risk but not having any symptoms; some progress through to experiencing symptoms requiring intervention but lack clarity for a syndromal diagnosis; this may move through to a first episode of the affective or psychotic disorder; and some then progress to experiencing recurrences or a chronic condition. In the later stages of the condition, effectiveness of usual treatments may decline, and may even be associated with worsening outcomes.[6] As in the case of many chronic physical illnesses where there may be limited potential for complete clinical recovery, treatment goals will not only focus on recovery from acute exacerbations and ongoing symptoms management, but also need to be tailored to the individual and the stage of the ill-health[6] and consider optimising or maintaining social and functional outcomes.

Regardless of illness course or stage, changes that occur as a result of SMHP (or even being considered 'at risk' of such conditions) can be confusing and frightening. There is uncertainty around the cause of the problem and the nature and effectiveness of potential treatments. People experiencing SMHP describe a number of important losses, including their sense of self and previous identity, which can become replaced with a focus on deficit and dysfunction.[7] Self-esteem, self-efficacy and sense of competence can become eroded, which may in turn increase the negative impact of the conditions, exacerbated by ongoing personal and public stigma and discrimination.[8,9] Established roles can be lost and individuals might lose:

> jobs
> relationships with partners
> relatives and friends
> custody of children.

The development of future plans and new potential roles become more challenging. 'Normal' milestones of adult development, such as:

> developing independence
> forming and maintaining intimate relationships
> choosing and following a career path
> developing new skills and hobbies

may be compromised, depending on the age at which ill-health presents. Challenges finding and maintaining employment can result in financial hardship or dependence. Demoralisation, the experience of hopelessness, helplessness and a loss of meaning and purpose in life[10] (see *Palliative Care within Mental Health: principles and philosophy*, Chapter 7) may result as a consequence of:

> ongoing stigma and multiple losses
> eroded self-esteem
> isolation
> loneliness
> limited social supports
> adverse treatment experiences.

Hopelessness is in turn associated with poor outcomes in physical and mental health problems.[10]

> **KEY POINT 10.1**

Families of people experiencing SMHP are often their primary support.

Family members may take a role as a primary carer if necessary, providing instrumental support such as:

➤ assisting with activities of daily living
➤ providing financial support
➤ staying actively involved
➤ providing a sense of belonging, emotional support and affection.

Family members are not immune to the effects of stigma, either suffering the consequences of public stigma or having their own behaviours affected by stereotypes and assumptions. Further, as with any chronic ill-health, the caring role impacts on the carer's:

➤ mental health
➤ quality of life
➤ well-being
➤ physical health.

It has been well established that the physical health of people experiencing SMHP is poorer than the general community. People experiencing SMHP experience greater rates of:

➤ obesity
➤ metabolic syndrome
➤ diabetes mellitus
➤ cardiovascular disease

as well as more chronic viral infections and respiratory diseases than the general community.[11] Further, frequently two or more mental health conditions co-occur, and substance use problems (*see* Chapter 14) are common in people experiencing SMHP.[12,13] Such comorbidity can negatively impact on treatment outcomes.[14]

PALLIATIVE CARE AND LONG-TERM MENTAL HEALTH

In SMHP, treatment goals often mirror those of chronic physical ill-health; with a focus on increasing or maintaining functioning while recognising the limited capacity for complete resolution of the disorder. 'Recovery' in SMHP can refer to clinical, social and functional improvements, as well as experiencing a better life despite having the condition, rather than complete recovery as seen for acute medical conditions.[3] The World Health Organization defines palliative care as:

> an approach that improves the quality of life of patients and their families facing the problems associated with life-threatening illness, through the prevention and relief of suffering by means of early identification and impeccable assessment and treatment of pain and other problems, physical, psychosocial and spiritual.[15]

The palliative care approach, rather than focusing on complete resolution of the ill-health, aims to provide relief from distressing symptoms, offers support to the individual and family to assist with coping and living life as actively as possible in the face of persistent symptoms and disability, and provides an intra- inter-disciplinary approach to address needs of individual and their families, including coping with losses and redefining goals of care.[15] It can be applied to diverse populations, and is particularly relevant to the needs of people experiencing SMHP, their families and those caring for them.

KEY POINT 10.2

Palliative care is appropriate at any point during serious ill-health, and can be delivered alongside treatments targeting symptoms and clinical recovery.

It has been argued that for people experiencing treatment-resistant ill-health, the palliative care model is a more appropriate treatment approach than traditional symptom-focused approaches that may not be providing any benefits and may be potentially causing harm.[16] Nevertheless, in doing so, it is critical that appropriate assessment of remediable factors contributing to so-called treatment resistance are reviewed and addressed, and the risk of inappropriate therapeutic pessimism is carefully scrutinised, especially given the stigma of hopelessness that can distort the care of people experiencing schizophrenia.

In this chapter we present three case studies of people experiencing long-term mental health conditions. These case studies are set within a general medical hospital setting and will be used to highlight and discuss common challenges faced by individuals experiencing SMHP, their families and supports, and professionals. The cases will also illustrate how the principles underlying palliative care approaches can be applied when working alongside people experiencing SMHP.

Case Study 10.1 – Mark – Part I

Mark (48) is a security guard who had been living in his car for the past two weeks after his wife threw him out. He was admitted to the orthopaedic ward to treat a compound fracture of his elbow, sustained when he lost control of his motorbike while speeding around a corner.

Nursing staff noted that he was irritable and spoke so quickly that he was hard to understand. They also described him as 'full of himself' and 'annoying' because he used his call button frequently, did not sleep and was disturbing other people with his 'stories'.

Mark was referred for a mental health assessment. He reported feeling very well and whilst he acknowledged that doctors had labelled him with a diagnosis of bipolar affective disorder 20 years ago, he was adamant that this was a mistake. He had been admitted to a mental health unit twice previously, at 23 and 36 years of age, and stated that he had been forced by a court order to take medications that had no benefit and caused bad side effects. As soon as the court order relapsed he ceased the medication and had not had any psychotropic medications for the past five years.

Mental state examination revealed a thin, somewhat dishevelled man, dressed in street clothes and with a large bandage covering his right arm. He was distractible and restless, pacing by the side of his bed. His speech was pressured and difficult to interrupt, with loud volume. Whilst he said he felt fine he appeared to be irritable and suspicious. He showed flight of ideas and was preoccupied with leaving the hospital to move his car. He was sure his arm would be fine and wanted to drive several hundred kilometres to stay with his daughter. He stated several times that he was a highly trained security guard and could do a much better job than the hospital security staff who were on standby at the nurses' station. There were no delusions or hallucinations and he had limited insight into his physical and mental health problems.

REFLECTIVE PRACTICE EXERCISE 10.1

Time: 15 minutes

Mark was distressed and agitated and desperately trying to maintain a sense of dignity and control in an escalating situation. The nurses' comments that he is 'annoying' indicate that the professionals are struggling to accept the presence of someone with serious mental health problems in the acute surgical unit.

- Think about what factors affect your ability to care for people experiencing a mental health problem.
- Consider your own attitudes, beliefs and behaviours.

'THEY DO NOT FIT IN HERE'!

People experiencing chronic or co-occurring conditions are often seen within acute health services, or in services with a medical model approach, who can struggle when working with a person experiencing more complex needs. In a qualitative study, people experiencing SMHP seen in a general hospital setting reported finding themselves labelled; this label affecting how they were viewed by others as well as themselves.[17] They felt they were being judged negatively and treated differently, as well as often being ignored. Professionals' reports supported these beliefs.[17] In interviews with professionals working in general hospital settings with experiences managing people experiencing SMHP in general hospitals, several themes consistently emerge:[17,18]

➤ Staff struggle in an environment that is not conducive to delivery of the type of care they perceive is required. Challenges of this environment include a lack of time, the usual chaos that is present in a hospital ward and high levels of stimulation.

➤ Professionals perceive that they lack adequate knowledge and skills to work effectively alongside people experiencing serious and enduring mental health problems. This increases the stress they experience when they are then in the position of caring for the person. Professionals in general can describe experiencing fear, anxiety and uncertainty in relation to mental health problems and its consequences.

➤ Being trained and working within an acute care model, where full recovery is the goal, can make it difficult when working with people experiencing a chronic SMHP, who frequently reattend the service with the same problems. It can result in staff feeling hopeless and pessimistic for the person, and can be emotionally demanding.

➤ The stigma of mental health problems can result not only in fear and pessimism, but can also result in silence and avoidance, where communication is not attempted and care is not delivered or is different to that provided to others.

➤ SMHP may not be seen as a genuine condition; the person may be perceived as not belonging in the service and may be perceived as exaggerating physical symptoms.

The negative consequences of the effects of stigma on the care of the person experiencing SMHP can be prevented via:

➤ the professional working to address their own stereotypes and assumptions

➤ empathy for the person and the situation they are in and awareness of the persons vulnerability and dependence on the system of care they find themselves in, and the potential for this system of care to undermine an individual's identity or sense of self

➤ fostering dignity and hope using person-centred communication; getting to know and treat the individual as a whole person rather than the focus being on deficit and dysfunction; and focusing on what can be done, in order to maintain hope

➤ adequate training for professionals in the skills to communicate and respond effectively to common mental health problems and the mental health needs of the individual. This can improve the confidence of the health professional, improve attitudes to mental health problems, and improve person-centred care, especially if allied to ready access to supportive mental health professionals as needed.

DEVELOPMENT OF A THERAPEUTIC RELATIONSHIP

The effectiveness of any person–professional interaction relies heavily on a positive therapeutic relationship. In qualitative interviews with people experiencing SMHP the factors that the individual sees as important in establishing a therapeutic relationship support classical theories (e.g. see Rogers 1942, Yalom 1980 and Jung 1967, as cited in Shattell *et al.*, 2007)[19]. Core themes include:

➤ being alongside the individual, demonstrating empathy and respect and validating the person and their situation and concerns

➤ taking time to get to know the whole person (rather than as a diagnosis or stereotype); allowing the person to be an individual and treating her or him as a unique individual worthy of care; individualising care and sharing the power in the relationship

➤ being authentic; being honest and admitting what they do not know
➤ being skilled and professional; being prepared and having a plan; helping the person to find a solution to current problems (via education, appropriate referrals, recommended reference materials – *see* Chapter 15).

Respect for the:
➤ individual
➤ their beliefs
➤ their culture
➤ their desires
➤ their experiences
➤ their reference group (*see* Chapter 4)

is a core principle underlying the palliative care approach and arguably essential to all healthcare. An appreciation of the personal meaning of ill-health and its symptoms to the individual and family members with regard for their life experience, values, goals and personal expectations is just as relevant among people experiencing mental health problems, yet frequently unaddressed. Not being treated with respect or understanding, and feeling a burden to others, are the most commonly identified factors that people receiving palliative care believe influence their sense of dignity. 'Dignity-conserving care'[20,21] encourages the professional to examine their attitudes towards the person, which may be influenced by internal stereotypes or assumptions, and the impact of these on care provided.

KEY POINT 10.3

Health professionals are guided to ensure their behaviours are based on respect and kindness; to use person-centred communication strategies, aiming to get to know the whole person and their story; and to develop an understanding of the suffering of the person and the desire to relieve it.

Case Study 10.1 – Mark – Part II

When the psychiatrist arrived on the ward he was struck by the high degree of anxiety and tension among the staff who were hovering in the corridor. He asked Mark if he would mind moving back to his bed in a single room so that they could speak in privacy and lessen extraneous noise. The psychiatrist kept the door open to maintain a ready exit but sat down to interview Mark at eye level. He was mindful of Mark's hostility but tried to be as open as possible, explaining why he had been called to see Mark and what the treating team's concerns were. He was careful not to challenge or confront Mark's beliefs about his ill-health but worked hard at negotiating a plan of action that acknowledged Mark's own concerns but would also keep him safe.

TREATMENT ADHERENCE

Case Study 10.1 – Mark – Part III

Despite his best efforts, the psychiatrist was unable to establish an effective thera-peutic relationship with Mark. Considerable time was spent focusing on Mark's concerns about being labelled with a mental ill-health diagnosis and his anger about the psychiatrist's decision to prescribe an antipsychotic medication – olanzapine. Mark said that olanzapine did not do anything except 'bomb him out'.

For many individuals experiencing SMHP, medication is presented as the domi-nant treatment tool to manage symptoms. While people experiencing SMHP have described medication as a safety net to protect them from relapse and re-hospitalisation, and many see it as important, they also see recovery as no longer needing to take medication.[22,23,24]

While medication adherence is poor among people experiencing SMHP,[25] in gen-eral low rates of adherence to medication is the norm, across all people experiencing chronic conditions. The World Health Organization estimated that around 50% of people in developed countries with chronic diseases adhere to recommended treat-ment regimes, with rates potentially even lower in developing countries.[26] Even so, the 'normality' of not taking medication as recommended is generally not acknowl-edged, and people are labelled as non-compliant or difficult. Reasons behind not adhering to recommended treatments are complex, varied and multifactorial, with therapeutic alliance and communication playing a role in addition to individual and systems factors.[27] Development of a therapeutic relationship and eliciting the person's beliefs around their medications and their personal reasons for not following rec-ommendations will aid in developing joint treatment goals around medication use. Interventions targeting adherence uses shared decision making, and training packages that provide mental health professionals with adherence therapy skills may potentially lead to improved clinical outcomes for people experiencing SMHP.[25]

IMPACT AND ETHICS OF INVOLUNTARY TREATMENTS (*SEE* CHAPTER 3)

Case Study 10.1 – Mark – Part IV

Mark gave permission for the psychiatrist to speak with his daughter to obtain some collateral history. The daughter described a four-week deterioration in his mood and an increase in impulsive behaviours that had followed increasing arguments and an eventual separation from his second wife of 10 years. Mark had been send-ing incomprehensible text messages to his daughter and work colleagues and two days before the accident he had failed to attend work. The family had been unable to locate him because he had been living in his car. Mark had never accepted his diagnosis and had never engaged well with healthcare professionals.

> The psychiatrist rated Mark's risk of harm to self as high (*see* Chapter 9). He denied suicidal ideation or thoughts of harming others, but his manic state, limited insight, refusal of treatment, recent serious accident in which speed was a contributing factor and ongoing desire to drive with an immobilised arm all reinforced this viewpoint.
>
> Whilst shared decision making is ideal, Mark's lack of ill-health awareness, poor insight into his need for medication and the professionals' concerns about his level of risk added weight to the psychiatrist's decision to enforce treatment.
>
> Mark's mental health continued to deteriorate despite his eventual acceptance of a mood stabiliser and antipsychotic medication. After surgical intervention for his elbow fracture he was admitted on an involuntary basis into the local mental health hospital.

Mark had the experience of having two forms of involuntary treatment administered – first the medication, and then the admission to mental health services. Person-centred care approaches emphasise the importance of a shared power base between the person and the health professional, and shared decision making. However, when a person's safety or physical health is at risk and that person is refusing treatment their wishes and decisions can be overruled if there are grounds to believe their decision making is affected by mental ill-health (for example, by invoking a Mental Health Act) or other condition affecting their capacity to make informed conditions (for example, medical guardianship).

Involuntary treatment is an ethical and moral minefield (*see* Chapter 3). Further, for the person experiencing treatment, experiences and outcomes can vary. The individuals' perception of coercion during involuntary admission, as opposed to the professional's documentation of the extent of coercive measures, has been found to influence satisfaction with care during involuntary admissions.[28] This suggests that for the person, feelings of coercion may depend more on the overall manner in which treatment is delivered, negotiated and explained.[28] Interviews with people who have experienced involuntary admissions highlight values to be considered by the mental health professional in this situation,[29] including:

➤ freedom of choice
➤ feeling safe
➤ non-paternalistic and respectful behaviour from professionals.

Overall, even in the case of involuntary treatment, when the person believes their best interests have been kept in mind, their opinions are being heard and taken into account, and they are still participating in their own care, satisfaction with care is increased.[28]

REFLECTIVE PRACTICE EXERCISE 10.2

Time: 20 minutes

Find your local legal legislations that may be enacted to enforce involuntary treatment (for example Mental Health Acts, guardianship, etc.).

Consider:

- How could you work to maintain a therapeutic relationship where involuntary treatment is required?
- How could you minimise loss of dignity and respect in a situation where involuntary treatment is required?

KEY POINT 10.4

The need to enforce treatment is inevitable in some high-risk situations but it is important to work with the individual as much as possible and to always consider less restrictive treatment options.

Case Study 10.2 – Maria – Part I

Maria (52) is a single woman experiencing chronic schizophrenia who is living with her elderly mother. Her father died five years ago; her brother and sister have limited contact with her because they live a considerable distance away and are 'involved in their own lives'. Fellow church members provide some social support. In her twenties and thirties, Maria had many admissions to mental health hospitals for distressing exacerbations of her psychosis. At times these lasted as long as 12 months. However, in the past 10 years, since she has been taking clozapine, her mental health has improved to the point where she has had no further admissions, and the local community mental health team has handed her care back to her family doctor and closed the service request.

While Maria has avoided admissions she has never been symptom-free. She experiences intermittent auditory hallucinations with a voice providing a running commentary of her actions, particularly when she is feeling anxious. Although she has developed some strategies to cope with these, including listening to music and singing songs, she also has prominent negative symptoms that are very disabling. These include social withdrawal and anhedonia. She has little interest in social activities outside a weekly visit to church and has a limited repertoire of daily activities. Her mother has always done the shopping, cooking and cleaning while Maria watches television or sits in the garden.

Maria has put on 40 kilograms in weight in the past few years and has developed diabetes and hypertension. Her family doctor has encouraged her to increase her level of physical activity, but her amotivation, weight and progressive knee osteoarthritis have limited this.

Maria was admitted to the local hospital for a knee replacement and was referred to the mental health team the day after her operation because she was mumbling to herself and the professionals were concerned that she was experiencing an exacerbation of her schizophrenia.

MEDICAL HEALTH VERSUS MENTAL HEALTH

Despite being at higher risk of co-occurring physical ill-health, evidence suggests that people experiencing SMHP are less likely to receive appropriate screening and care for physical ill-health, and quality of care has been found to be inferior to that provided to those with no comparable mental disorder.[30] For example, although depression is an established psychosocial risk factor for coronary heart disease, people experiencing a charted history of depression attending an emergency department with an acute myocardial infarction were more likely to receive a low-priority triage score and miss benchmark time for key screening and treatment procedures compared to people experiencing other comorbidities.[31]

There are a number of potential reasons behind this discrepancy in care. Misdiagnosis may occur, with physical health symptoms being attributed to mental health or substance use (drug and alcohol) issues. External stigma, discomfort or lack of confidence on the part of the health professional may result in treatment refusal or adjustment. Symptoms of the mental health condition itself (for example, thought disorder in chronic schizophrenia) may impede clear communication of concerns or problems to health professionals. The individual may avoid presenting to clinical services with problematic symptoms due to discomfort, internalised stigma or past negative experiences. Conversely, the person and/or their family may overcome real or perceived service barriers by engaging in less appropriate behaviours to get the person medical attention, potentially increasing existing tension between the individual and the professional.

In the case of acute ill-health, whether an exacerbation of the SMHP, co-occurring physical health issue, or both, a common problem is the tendency for all changes in the person's mental health to be attributed to mental ill-health. In order to avoid potential misdiagnosis it is important to conduct a thorough assessment that is not biased by assumptions and stereotypes (*see* Chapter 7). Having detailed information about the person's baseline functioning will aid in determining whether symptoms described are new, pre-existing or previously experienced, and whether behaviour and cognitive state is more or less usual for that person. This highlights the importance of seeking collateral information where possible.

Case Study 10.2 – Maria – Part II

On further assessment, the ward doctor noted that Maria was agitated and frightened. She had not slept the previous night. She was disorientated to time, place and person and appeared to be responding to visual hallucinations, pointing at something on the bed sheets and mumbling about cats. Her attention and concentration were poor and she refused to answer direct questions from staff. Maria's mother confirmed that her symptoms were different from those that had precipitated mental health admissions, and described her as 'really muddled and confused'. She also pointed out that Maria had been 'absolutely fine' before her operation.

After mental health review Maria's treating team reluctantly accepted that she had a post-operative delirium rather than 'a psychiatric problem'. A thorough physical examination and laboratory tests revealed normal vital signs, a slightly elevated white cell count and a stable clozapine level but no other clear aetiological factors. The delirium settled over the next few days with non-pharmacological interventions that included environmental and clinical care strategies and regular emotional support by Maria's mother, who was more effective at soothing Maria's agitation than the health professionals (*see* Chapter 5).

FAMILY AND SUPPORT SYSTEMS

Case Study 10.2 – Maria – Part III

During one of her hospital visits, Maria's mother revealed to a nurse that she had just turned 86. She commented that while she was remarkably fit and active for her age, she was worried about Maria's future: 'who will look after her when I'm gone'?

Palliative care guidelines provide specific recommendations for working with family members that are directly applicable to the mental health setting.[32] A particular family member of a person experiencing SMHP may become a long-term primary carer. Carers of people experiencing any chronic ill-health are at increased risk of stress, 'burnout', depression and other forms of emotional distress, and physical problems.[33] Considering the needs and impact of the situation on the family is vital to help prevent or minimise these negative consequences. Strategies include:[32]

➤ checking with the person who their primary supports are (whether family or others) and their preferences around the involvement of those people in their care and decision making
➤ after gaining approval from the person, gathering information from identified support people as part of the assessment process, and considering how they can be involved in planning and decision making around treatment, rehabilitation or care processes. At the same time, be aware of and consider the culture and cultural preferences of identified support people as a part of this process (*see* Chapter 4)
➤ monitoring the needs of support people. Be aware that these may change over time, possibly quickly, as such mechanisms need to be flexible and responsive
➤ support strategies may aim to help the family or support person provide effective care, for example education, problem-solving assistance and practical supports

➤ other strategies target the carer directly, including highlighting to the carer the importance of caring for their own health, and providing options to assist in this process

➤ strategies targeting carer burden include respite care, available frequently and in case of emergency.

KEY POINT 10.5

Good communication between all parties is vital (*see* Chapter 15).

Case Study 10.2 – Maria – Part IV

With Maria's permission a family conference was scheduled to explore in more depth the role of the family in Maria's treatment and rehabilitation, the nature of her relationship with her family, the overall family functioning and the impact of Maria's behaviour and ill-health on her family.

It emerged that Maria was the youngest of three children. The first signs of psychosis had appeared in her late teens, and her mother, who had always been protective of her 'little girl', was keen to shelter her from a mental health diagnosis with its associated stigma. The older siblings had left home and pursued their own careers and relationships, and while there was no overt disharmony in the family, Maria's mother wondered if they stayed away because they were scared of Maria's schizophrenia diagnosis. Maria's mother had never worked and said she had always been happy looking after Maria. The father was a 'good provider' but had never been very involved in Maria's mental health problems or treatments. The mother stated that, in retrospect, she may have been too protective; she had wanted to keep Maria away from the mental health system but now realised that the system may have been able to help prepare Maria for independent living in the community. There were no other family members who could help.

RECOVERY AND PLANNING FOR THE FUTURE

As with Maria, many people experiencing SMHP experience ongoing symptoms even when medical treatment is stabilised. However, even when medical treatment is unchanged, there remains scope for people experiencing SMHP to experience further clinical, functional and social improvements. Concepts including wellness, recovery and self-management are being taken up, particularly in the area of chronic disease, and can potentially lead to further improvements by virtue of being health-centred rather than disease-centred. In these approaches, the individual plays a central role in managing their health and healthcare, and there is an acknowledgement that a person can maintain wellness while experiencing an ongoing health condition.[34] The person is a shared decision-maker with equal power in the relationship. This is different to a paternalistic or directive medical model, where decision making is left to the health professionals, and the 'patient's job' is to comply. Where treatment approaches are collaborative, with all parties working together, and communicating, there is greater opportunity for the individual's needs to be met, and to ensure there are no gaps or inconsistencies in treatment approaches.

Advance directives, instructions outlining the person's wishes regarding treatment in the case of future incapacity, have often been used with regard to mental health care by people experiencing SMHP, but less so for future medical care.[35] Interviews with people experiencing SMHP indicate that while a quarter had thought about treatment preferences in the case of becoming seriously medically ill, few had discussed them with anyone, even though 72% believed someone should make medical health care decisions for a person who is unable to.[35] Palliative care guidelines strongly recommend such future planning with the individual,[32] both in the case of a crisis and of end-of-life care (*see* Chapter 6, *Palliative Care within Mental Health: principles and philosophy*, Chapters 13 and 14). In addition to the individual's wishes and preferences, plans should take into account cultural preferences, be well documented, identify the support needs of the carer, care workers and volunteers, identify other available support staff, and ensure the family knows who to contact in event of a change or crisis.

Case Study 10.2 – Maria – Part V

The current admission for a knee replacement provided an excellent opportunity for clinicians to re-evaluate Maria's complex care needs. However, the acute surgical team was reluctant to prolong her admission. Maria's delirium and the prominent negative symptoms of schizophrenia had already slowed her recovery and extended her stay in the acute unit, so she was transferred to a rehabilitation ward for ongoing care.

From the outset the rehabilitation team noted that Maria had not been very involved in defining her own needs and goals. Her mother or treating professionals had always spoken or acted on her behalf and whilst their intentions were well-meaning, Maria had been given very little opportunity to collaborate in her recovery process.

A care co-ordinator was allocated to Maria, and while her physical rehabilitation proceeded, the team began the complex process of assessing her needs. Perhaps because of her negative symptoms, Maria found it difficult to maintain enthusiasm for this process. Her mother identified primarily the need for improving independent living skills. Maria thought that she might like to increase her social activities and her physicians highlighted her poor physical health, placing emphasis on her need for weight loss and increased exercise. She was already attending monthly medical reviews with her family doctor for clozapine monitoring, but the local specialist mental health service had withdrawn their care, closing off any opportunities for involvement in supported recovery programmes or peer support groups.

Re-establishing contact with the community mental health team was identified as the first priority. The team agreed to provide case management to monitor and treat mental health problems, supervise the recovery process, ensure good communication between external health professionals who would help with independent living skills and to work closely with the family doctor so that Maria's physical health needs were not neglected. A case conference, which included Maria, her mother and the key case professional, was held before Maria's discharge. Maria's care plan was documented and dates set for regular case planning and needs reassessment.

KEY POINT 10.6

- In a general medical setting, a person who has been labelled in the past with a mental health disorder is at increased risk of undetected physical ill-health.
- Actively seek collateral history to establish baseline level of functioning and identify subtle changes in symptom presentation.
- For people experiencing serious mental health problems, families and friends play an important support role.
- Always seek the person's consent before interviewing family members.
- Families have needs too.
- An integrated community care plan works best if there is a fixed point of responsibility for implementation and clear communication lines between professionals, the individual and their social support system.
- Care plans need to be flexible to reflect the person's changing choices and needs.

Case Study 10.3 – Anna – Part I

Anna (24) is a single woman who was admitted to the Intensive Care Unit after swallowing drain cleaner in a suicide attempt while intoxicated with alcohol (*see* Chapters 9, 14). Her mother reported that Anna had recently broken up with her boyfriend. She had a long history of self-harm attempts with self-cutting and self-poisoning and had been diagnosed with a borderline personality disorder. She was currently engaged in a psychotherapy treatment programme (Dialectical Behaviour Therapy)[36] and before the relationship ended she had been managing well. The frequency of her cutting episodes had reduced, she had stopped binge drinking alcohol and for the last two months had been enjoying a new job as a waitress. She was not taking any psychotropic medication but had trialled antidepressants in the past without perceived benefit.

Unfortunately Anna's oesophageal burns were severe and carried a high risk of oesophageal perforation or strictures. In addition, she required a tracheostomy to counter laryngeal swelling, although doctors were hopeful that this would not be permanent.

When Anna regained consciousness she was able to describe the events leading to the suicide attempt. Initially she could only communicate by writing and she recorded: 'I was angry with Mike … it was so fucking stupid … I didn't really want to die.'

She regretted not using the emotion regulation skills that she had learned in therapy and was distressed about her physical injuries, which carried an uncertain prognosis.

Individuals experiencing a severe personality disorder are likely to have a difficult time in health settings, particularly the general hospital setting. Anna was comfortable with the diagnosis of borderline personality disorder because she felt the label had an explanatory power that helped her to understand the way she felt and behaved. However, for many health professionals, a personality disorder is an indicator that a person will be 'difficult', 'demanding' and 'manipulative'.

The general hospital environment creates further stress for these individuals. Communication lines are unclear and inconsistent, and very few treatments run to time.

From the outset it is important to maintain clear boundaries and develop a comprehensive care plan that identifies the person's needs and goals and specifies the role of each professional. Regular case conferences involving key professionals provide a useful forum for re-aligning the person's needs and care strategies as the admission proceeds.

Case Study 10.3 – Anna – Part II

Anna's care team consisted of the gastroenterology registrar and resident medical officer, who agreed to regularly update Anna on her physical progress and clearly explain and interpret the thoughts of the medical team about diagnosis and treatment; a senior ward nurse, whose role was to co-ordinate input from other professionals and act as a liaison between rotating ward nurses and Anna; an experienced mental health professional, who aimed to develop and model a supportive alliance with Anna, monitor and treat comorbid mental health conditions, assess and manage suicide risk, and be available to help professionals process their emotional reactions to Anna; and a dietician, who oversaw the complexities of Anna's nutritional needs given her pending gastrostomy. The healthcare team met regularly at weekly intervals in a case conference setting and while Anna was not present at these, the lead nurse always provided Anna with a summary of the discussion after each session.

Over the next three weeks Anna was distressed by the attitudes of two night nurses who were vocal about the fact that the injury was something that Anna had done to herself, but on the whole the admission progressed relatively smoothly. Regular, consistent communication amongst professionals (*see* Chapter 15), the active inclusion of Anna in all treatment decisions and the use of firm limits around problematic behaviours by Anna and negative comments by professionals ensured that Anna was able to manage her distressing ill-health experience, and the healthcare team were left with a sense of collaboration and professionalism.

SELF-CARE FOR HEALTH PROFESSIONALS

In any role within the caring profession, we all need to ensure there are strategies in place for our own self-care to minimise risk of burnout. Reflective practice, the process of paying attention to and reflecting on antecedents and consequences of behaviours, can help to identify beliefs and assumptions that are influencing reactions to situations. Identifying and addressing these 'triggers' can result in behaviour change that can lead to better communication and therapeutic alliance with the person experiencing SMHP. This may then lead to decreased stress for the health professional. Reflective practice can be enhanced by supportive supervision or mentoring relationships with an experienced peer (*see* Chapter 15).[37] Some situations may provoke reactions due to similarities with the health professionals' lived experiences, leading to over-identification or retraumatisation. Mentoring and/or counselling for the health professional can help in these situations. Engaging supports within or external to the healthcare team, can bring in additional skills and approaches that may assist in managing difficult situations. Finally, health professionals can also follow guidelines provided for carers, with regard to prioritising their own health and taking time out as needed.

KEY POINT 10.7

- All health clinicians have values and beliefs that may affect their therapeutic relationship with the individual.
- All professionals will have a range of emotional responses to each individual and it is important to understand these rather than react to them.

SUMMARY AND CONCLUSIONS

Mark, Maria and Anna's stories are all unique. However, several common themes emerge that are not only relevant to their situation but for many experiencing SMHP. Emerging themes include the experience of stigma and its detrimental impact on care; the importance of communication and therapeutic alliance in the development and delivery of care plans; the impact of the ill-health, treatment and healthcare system on their family and loved ones; and the importance of assessing, understanding and respecting the individual's opinions, concerns, values, culture (*see* Chapter 4) and spirituality (see *Palliative Care within Mental Health: principles and philosophy*, Chapter 8) during treatment planning, delivery and beyond.

KEY POINT 10.8

Functional and social recovery can be hindered by a focus on acute symptom assessment and management rather than the person-centred experience and needs of the individual.

The palliative care approach, with a focus on the whole person, living life and coping in the face of serious life problems, can provide professionals with (working alongside people experiencing SMHP) extra tools and strategies to ensure quality, person-centred healthcare for each individual and their family.

REFERENCES

1 Kessler RC, Aguilar-Gaxiola S, Alonso J, *et al.* The global burden of mental disorders: an update from the WHO World Mental Health (WMH) Surveys. *Epidemiologia e Psichiatria Sociale.* 2011; **18**: 23–33.

2 Wang PS, Aguilar-Gaxiola S, Alonso J, *et al.* Use of mental health services for anxiety, mood, and substance disorders in 17 countries in the WHO world mental health surveys. *Lancet.* 2007; **370**: 841–50.

3 Jaaskelainen E, Juola P, Hirvonen N, *et al.* A systematic review and meta-analysis of recovery in schizophrenia. *Schizophrenia Bulletin.* 2013; **39**: 1296–306.

4 McGorry PD, Hickie IB, Yung AR, *et al.* Clinical staging of psychiatric disorders: a heuristic framework for choosing earlier, safer and more effective interventions. *Australian and New Zealand Journal of Psychiatry.* 2006; **40**: 616–22.

5 Trauer T. Palliative models of care for later stages of mental disorder: maximising recovery, maintaining hope and building morale. *Australian and New Zealand Journal of Psychiatry.* 2012; **46**: 170–2.

6 Berk M, Brnabic A, Dodd S, *et al.* Does stage of illness impact treatment response in bipolar disorder? Empirical treatment data and their implication for the staging model and early intervention. *Bipolar Disorder.* 2011; **13**: 87–98.

7 Wisdom JP, Bruce K, Saedi GA, *et al.* 'Stealing me from myself': identity and recovery in personal accounts of mental illness. *Australian and New Zealand Journal of Psychiatry.* 2008; **42**: 489–95.

8 Sartorius N. Lessons from a 10-year global programme against stigma and discrimination because of an illness. *Psychology Health and Medicine.* 2006; **11**: 383–8.

9 Thornicroft G, Brohan E, Rose D, *et al.* Global pattern of experienced and anticipated discrimination against people with schizophrenia: a cross-sectional survey. *Lancet.* 2009; **373**: 408–15.

10 Clarke DM and Kissane DW. Demoralization: its phenomenology and importance. *Australian and New Zealand Journal of Psychiatry.* 2002; **36**: 733–42.

11 De Hert M, Correll CU, Bobes J, *et al.* Physical illness in patients with severe mental disorders. I. Prevalence, impact of medications and disparities in health care. *World Psychiatry.* 2011; **10**: 52–77.

12 Kessler RC, Chiu WT, Demler O, *et al.* Prevalence, severity, and comorbidity of 12-month DSM-IV disorders in the National Comorbidity Survey Replication. *Archives of General Psychiatry.* 2005; **62**: 617–27.

13 Havassy BE, Alvidrez J, Owen KK. Comparisons of patients with comorbid psychiatric and substance use disorders: implications for treatment and service delivery. *Amercian Journal of Psychiatry.* 2004; **161**: 139–45.

14 Johnson J. Cost-effectiveness of mental health services for persons with a dual diagnosis: a literature review and the CCMHCP. The Cost-Effectiveness of Community Mental Health Care for Single and Dually Diagnosed Project. *Journal of Substance Abuse Treatment.* 2000; **18**: 119–27.

15 World Health Organization. *WHO Definition of Palliative Care.* Available at: www.who.int/cancer/palliative/definition/en/ (accessed 11 December 2013).

16 Berk M, Berk L, Udina M, *et al.* Palliative models of care for later stages of mental disorder: maximizing recovery, maintaining hope, and building morale. *Australian and New Zealand Journal of Psychiatry.* 2012; **46**: 92–9.

17 Liggins J, Hatcher S. Stigma toward the mentally ill in the general hospital: a qualitative study. *General Hospital Psychiatry.* 2005; **27**: 359–64.

18 Marynowski-Traczyk D, Broadbent M. What are the experiences of Emergency Department nurses in caring for clients with a mental illness in the Emergency Department? *Australasian Emergency Nursing Journal.* 2001; **14**: 172–9.

19 Shattell MM, Starr SS, Thomas SP. 'Take my hand, help me out': mental health service recipients' experience of the therapeutic relationship. *International Journal of Mental Health Nursing.* 2007; **16**: 274–84.

20 Chochinov HM. Dignity-conserving care – a new model for palliative care: helping the patient feel valued. *Journal of the American Medical Association.* 2002; **287**: 2253–60.

21 Chochinov HM. Dignity and the essence of medicine: the A, B, C, and D of dignity conserving care. *British Medical Journal.* 2007; **335**: 184–7.

22 Piat M, Sabetti J, Bloom D. The importance of medication in consumer definitions of recovery from serious mental illness: a qualitative study. *Issues in Mental Health Nursing.* 2009; **30**: 482–90.

23 Sullivan W. A long and winding road: the process of recovery from severe mental illness. *Innovations and Research in Clinical Services, Community Support and Rehabilitation.* 1994; **3**: 19–27.

24 Svedberg B, Backenroth-Ohsako G, Lutzen K. On the path to recovery: patients' experiences of treatment with long-acting injections of antipsychotic medication. *International Journal of Mental Health Nursing.* 2003; **12**: 110–8.

25 Gray R, White J, Schulz M, *et al.* Enhancing medication adherence in people with schizophrenia: an international programme of research. *International Journal of Mental Health Nursing.* 2010; **19**: 36–44.

26 World Health Organization. *Adherence to Long-term Therapies: Evidence for Action.* Switzerland: World Health Organization; 2003.

27 Brown MT, Bussell JK. Medication adherence: WHO cares? *Mayo Clin Proceedings.* 2001; **86**: 304–14.

28 Katsakou C, Bowers L, Amos T, *et al.* Coercion and treatment satisfaction among involuntary patients. *Psychiatric Services.* 2010; **61**: 286–92.

29 Valenti E, Giacco D, Katasakou C, *et al.* Which values are important for patients during involuntary treatment? A qualitative study with psychiatric inpatients. *Journal of Medical Ethics.* 2013; Oct 15; Epub ahead of print; doi: 10.1136/medethics-2011-100370/.

30 Mitchell AJ, Malone D, Doebbeling CC. Quality of medical care for people with and without comorbid mental illness and substance misuse: systematic review of comparative studies. *British Journal of Psychiatry.* 2009; **194**: 491–9.

31 Atzema CL, Schull MJ, Tu JV. The effect of a charted history of depression on emergency department triage and outcomes in patients with acute myocardial infarction. *Canadian Medical Association Journal.* 2011; **183**: 663–9.

32 Australian Government Department of Health and Ageing. *Guidelines for a Palliative Approach for Aged Care in the Community Setting: best practice guidelines for the Australian context.* Canberra: Australian Government Department of Health and Ageing; 2011.

33 Schulz R, Beach SR. Caregiving as a risk factor for mortality: the Caregiver Health Effects Study. *Journal of the American Medical Association.* 1999; **282**: 2215–9.

34 Sterling EW, von Esenwein SA, Tucker S, *et al.* Integrating wellness, recovery, and self-management for mental health consumers. *Community Mental Health Journal.* 2010; **46**: 130–8.

35 Foti ME, Bartels SJ, Merriman MP, *et al.* Medical advance care planning for persons with serious mental illness. *Psychiatric Services.* 2005; **56**: 576–84.

36 Korman LM, Burns KME. The young person and dialectical behaviour therapy. In: Cooper DB, editor. *Practice in Mental Health–Substance Use.* London: Radcliffe Publishing; 2011. pp. 169–83.

37 Meier DE. The inner life of physicians and care of the seriously ill. *Journal of the American Medical Association.* 2001; **286**: 3007.

TO LEARN MORE

- Andreasen NC, editor. *Schizophrenia: from mind to molecule.* Washington, DC: American Psychiatric Press, Inc.; 1994.
- beyondblue, the national depression initiative, Australia. Available at: www.beyondblue.org.au (accessed 11 December 2013).
- Corrigan P. *On the Stigma of Mental Illness: practical strategies for research and social change.* Washington, DC: American Psychological Association; 2004.
- Cooper DB, Cooper J, editors. *Palliative Care within Mental Health: principles and philosophy.* London/New York: Radcliffe Publishing; 2012.
- Kleinman A. *The Illness Narratives: suffering, healing, and the human condition.* New York: Basic Books; 1988.
- Mind, for better mental health (UK). Available at: www.mind.org.uk (accessed 11 December 2013).
- National Institute of Mental Health (US). Available at: www.nimh.nih.gov/index.shtml (accessed 11 December 2013).
- National Institute for Health and Clinical Excellence (UK). *Mental Health and Behavioural Conditions Guidelines.* Available at: http://guidance.nice.org.uk/Topic/MentalHealthBehavioural (accessed 11 December 2013).
- SANE Australia. Available at: www.sane.org (accessed 11 December 2013).
- SANE UK. Available at: www.sane.org.uk (accessed 11 December 2013)
- The Lancet Global Mental Health Series, launched 3 September 2007. Available at: www.thelancet.com/series/global-mental-health# (accessed 11 December 2013).

CHAPTER 11

Dementia, Alzheimer's and confusion

Joyce Simard

INTRODUCTION

The number of cases of Alzheimer's disease (AD) or a related irreversible dementia sweeping the world has been referred to as a 'tsunami' because of the devastation, both financial and emotional, of the person experiencing dementia as well as their families. The end-of-life costs in the United States and in the United Kingdom (UK) are helping to bankrupt their healthcare systems.[1] In human terms, the impact of people experiencing advanced dementia spending the last days or weeks in a hospital setting or in an intensive care unit can only be described as costly and an inhuman way to die. A palliative care approach to end-of-life care for people experiencing dementia saves money and is a humanistic way to live and to die as quality of life, relieving without curing, are the goals throughout the disease process.

KEY POINT 11.1

Professionals and families often feel the need to 'do everything' to prolong life, but it often prolongs the dying, not the living.

Professionals must be part of another tsunami, one that helps families of people experiencing AD understand the benefits of a palliative care approach to managing an irreversible dementia and understand that at some point in the disease process the burdens of aggressive medical interventions will far outweigh the benefits.

One of the biggest challenges facing professionals counselling families of people experiencing AD or another irreversible dementia to accept a palliative approach to care, is that physicians rarely tell the family that AD is an irreversible, terminal disease and that medical decisions and goals of care change as the disease progresses. There are three possible goals of care:
1 prolongation of life
2 maintenance of function
3 comfort.[2]

Unfortunately, often it is not possible to accomplish all three goals and the goals have to be prioritised. For instance, if a person is hospitalised in an intensive care unit to assure prolongation of life, that person will lose function and not be comfortable. In the early stage of AD, the primary goal of care is prolongation of life and may involve hospitalisation. In the later stage of the disease, the primary goal of care may be comfort, and therefore the person would not be hospitalised.

The primary goals for three stages of dementia may be:

1 **Early stage–mild memory loss** – Prolongation of life – this may mean hospitalisation, surgery, rehabilitation, aggressive treatment of infections, tube feedings and resuscitation from a cardiac arrest.

2 **Middle stage–moderate memory loss** – Maintenance of function – at this stage of an irreversible dementia, hospitalisation may cause more burden than benefit for persons experiencing dementia. He or she does not understand the confusion, noise, shared rooms and may be restrained because she or he do not understand the need to stay in bed or in their rooms. Many studies show that a person in this stage of a dementing ill-health has better results when she or he is cared for in a nursing home instead of in a hospital.[3] Hospitalisation usually results in loss of function.[4]

3 **Late stage–severe memory loss** – Comfort – people experiencing advanced dementia are often in need of total care and rarely need aggressive medical treatment.

KEY POINT 11.2

The primary goal is relieving suffering both physical and emotional.

The Alzheimer's Society in the UK has produced a leaflet titled 'This is me'. There is a place on the front to insert the person's picture and the inside has information about the needs, interests, preferences, likes and dislikes of the person with memory loss, who may not be able to communicate effectively. It can be easily downloaded from www.alzheimers.org.uk/site/scripts/download_info.php?downloadID=399 (accessed 10 May 2014).

Deciding on the goals of care for a person experiencing dementia is far too often an unwanted burden thrust on families during a medical crisis because the person experiencing dementia no longer has the capacity to make these important decisions. Unfortunately, even though most people want to decide on end-of-life care, most do not have advanced directives in place, so it is left in the hands of others. In the United States, fewer than 20% of Americans have an advanced directive in place.[5] Yearly reports produced by The End-of-Life Strategy, a 10-year plan adopted in the United Kingdom in 2008, indicate a heightened public awareness of end-of-life issues[6] but a recognition that more needs to be done to educate the general public.

Professionals can help people with end-of-life discussions (*see* Chapter 6). However, some feel as if they do not have the proper skills to initiate this type of conversation.

Two new resources are available to educate the public in talking about end-of-life issues. In the United States, a new movement called Death Cafe (*see* http://deathcafe. com/what/) is helping people join with others in an informal setting where they 'eat cake, drink tea and discuss death. Our objective is to increase awareness of death with a veiw to helping people make the most of their [finite] lives'.

Another resource is a series of DVDs produced by two men in Wisconsin who lost loved ones to severe chronic disease and created a prize-winning film, *Consider the Conversation: a documentary on a taboo subject*. Their goal is to:

> inspire culture change that results in end-of-life care that is more person-centred and less system-centred.

Their second film, *Consider the Conversation 2: a documentary about unintended consequences* is about the person–doctor relationship and the communication that is so important to helping both parties navigate the murky waters of severe chronic disease like AD. Both of these resources can provide professionals with the resources they need to help educate the public on the importance of making end-of-life decisions before serious ill-health or an irreversible dementia robs the person of being able to make that decision themselves (see www.considertheconversation.org/about).

In my 35 years of working in the healthcare industry, I have seen a marked decrease in the number of people experiencing advanced dementia being tube fed and an increase in Do Not Resuscitate (DNR) orders. However, work remains on continuing to counsel families about futile medical interventions for people experiencing advanced dementia (*see* Chapters 3, 6 and 13).

In a long-term care setting, the nurses or social worker is the professional who often initiates the discussion about DNR orders, and who explains the futility of tube feeding. Although only one person is designated as the person who can make these medical decisions for the individual experiencing advanced dementia, he or she often comes under pressure from other family members, who might ask: 'Do you want to starve your mother?'

KEY POINT 11.3

As many family members as possible should be involved in end-of-life discussions.

With the internet services like Skype and conference calling, it is possible to have a family meeting even when the family's members live in other states, counties or even in other countries. Professionals can help change the paradigm of aggressive care until hospice care is appropriate by talking with the families about palliative care from the time of diagnosis (*see* Figure 11.1).

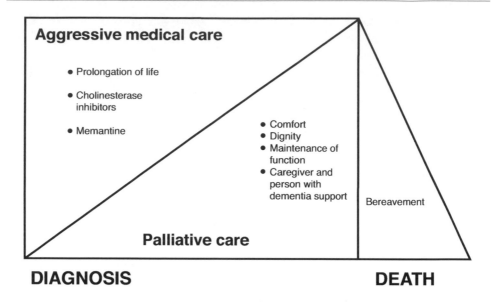

Figure 11.1 Stages of dementia from diagnosis to bereavement

EARLY STAGE OF DEMENTIA

Although current studies suggest that the median survival from initial diagnosis is 4.2 years for men and 5.7 years for women experiencing AD,[7] symptoms have probably been noticed by family members for 3 years before they actually go to a physician with complaints of memory loss and have a complete diagnostic workup. Far too often, the family dismisses memory loss as normal for an elderly person until a crisis occurs such as when father cannot find his way home from the local grocery store or mother leaves the stove on causing a fire.

Diagnosis

Professionals can help to educate the public to realise when memory loss begins to affect a person's ability to live independently; they need to see a physician, preferably a diagnostic centre specialising in AD. Unfortunately, the older person often fears the stigma of having a dementing disease and they are aware that there is no cure for AD. They deny that anything is wrong with them other than 'old age' until someone – their spouse, other family members or friends – realises the memory loss is more significant than just having 'senior moments'. People may not understand that there are reversible dementias that can be identified during the exam process.

KEY POINT 11.4

Current medications that appear to help some people experiencing memory loss are most effective taken in an early stage of a dementing illness.

Case Study 11.1 – Doris

Doris (76) had been retired for several years. She played golf with her husband and was in a women's golf league and she and her husband continued to host all major holidays for their six children and grandchildren, often feeding over 20 people at Christmas. Her favourite hobby was quilting and she joined her friends in a quilting club several times a month. Doris's children did not notice any significant problems with their mother's memory and if she did not remember something, they just thought it was a sign of normal ageing. Her husband gradually took on many of the tasks his wife was usually responsible for. Both Doris and her husband were in denial that she had the beginning of a serious memory problem. One day her daughter received a call from a member of the quilting club asking to meet her for coffee. When the daughter arrived, several women from the group were there and proceeded to tell her how worried they were about Doris. Doris was becoming increasingly frustrated with quilting, something she had done for years. She could not figure out where to place the squares and her sewing skills had deteriorated. They were all very concerned, as Doris was threatening to leave the group after so many years. The daughter was shocked and went to visit her father who after hearing about the quilters' concerns admitted that he too was worried. With the support of their children, Doris went to a diagnostic clinic, was diagnosed with probable AD, and was put on medication with good results from the treatment. Her quilting group helps her with quilting tasks and drives her to and from the club, and her children now host the major holiday celebrations. Doris is less frustrated and often jokes about her memory loss. Doris and her husband are relieved that the problem is now out in the open and they have chosen to live a full life in spite of the diagnosis.

In this early stage of a dementing disease, prolongation of life is the goal and hospitalisation may be appropriate, as in the case of a man with early memory loss who fell and broke his hip.

Case Study 11.2 – George

George (82) fell down the stairs and broke his hip. His physician thought that he was in the early stage of Alzheimer's disease, but with cueing and memory cards, he could follow directions. George did have surgery and, with a stay in a rehabilitation facility that understood his memory loss, he eventually could walk using a walker. He loved walking around the house and going to a favourite restaurant at least once a week. George was a happy man, tottering around with a colourful walker decorated by his grandchildren that was hard to forget! He continued to enjoy simple card games, reading his paper and other activities that he found enjoyable. Many activities were adapted so they were 'no fail'; he did not realise this and felt that he could continue activities that had always pleased him. His wife continued to help him feel that he was a help to her by asking his advice and reminding him with a smile that he still had jobs such as setting the table and wiping the dishes; these are the retirement jobs he had been doing for many years. His self-worth was validated and he was a happy man.

Spiritual life

In the early stage of AD, if a person is religious they still may be able to attend church services, although it is always best if a person who can help them remember names and guide them through the service accompanies them. As the disease progresses the confusion of attending church services may cause the person experiencing dementia more anxiety than staying home and watching a service on television. Some clergy will pay home visits to people experiencing dementia, and often churches have volunteers who might visit and even stay with the person so that the caregiver can do errands and have some time for themselves.

In the United States, we have celebrities who have announced that they have AD, and this has helped to humanise the disease. Ronald Regan's famous letter to the American public is one example:

> My fellow Americans, I have recently been told that I am one of the millions of Americans who will be afflicted with Alzheimer's disease. … So now we feel it is important to share it with you. In opening our hearts, we hope this might promote greater awareness of this condition. Perhaps it will encourage a clear understanding of the individuals and families who are affected by it. … I now begin the journey that will lead me into the sunset of my life. (see http://en.wikipedia.org/wiki/Ronald_Reagan).

He lived for 10 years after the letter was written and from all accounts lived life to its fullest for as long as possible, even riding his beloved horses for many years in spite of AD. This letter resulted in putting a face on AD and made it somewhat less of a stigma, especially for men.

President Reagan was very affectionate with his wife Nancy and in most pictures of them together they are holding hands. In this early stage, sexuality should not be a problem for people with AD, it may be that showing affection is as just as satisfying as ever, especially when it affects a senior who has had a lower sex drive, and intercourse may be more difficult to engage in. Counselling couples on alternative ways of making love can help relieve anxiety and maintain a close relationship in spite of the memory problems.

Sexuality

When someone experiences early onset dementia, before the age of 65, or a frontal lobe dementia the well spouse may have significant difficulty with having a satisfying sexual relationship for the remaining part of their marriage. Counselling or talking to others in a support group may help through this difficult time. There are currently

200,000 people experiencing early onset of dementia in the United States – see www. alz.org/alzheimers_disease_early_onset.asp – and 17,000 in the United Kingdom – see www.alzheimers.org.uk/site/scripts/documents_info.php?documentID=164.

Keeping people experiencing early memory loss in good mental health involves helping them feel needed, and involved in activities that have been in the past meaningful and pleasurable. It is easy to do things for people with memory loss, and that often results in them becoming dependent and depressed. They sense that something is wrong and they are not to be trusted to make decisions. In all aspects of their lives, the person should be asked to do as much for him- or herself as possible, choosing what to wear, helping with household chores and continuing hobbies. Adaptations need to be made as the disease progresses.

SELF-ASSESSMENT EXERCISE 11.1 (*SEE* ANSWERS ON P. 186)

Time: 20 minutes
- **Driving** – Driving is usually the 'man's job'. It has been determined that David is not safe to drive. How can his wife take over the driving responsibility and yet have him feel as if he is still in control?
- **Dressing** – Sara chooses a totally inappropriate outfit for church. How do you get her to change clothes without making her feel as if her choice was wrong for the occasion?
- **Playing cards** – Aileen has always enjoyed playing bridge but now cannot figure out how to follow the rules of play. What alternatives can be suggested?

Communication

When a person experiences dementia, even in the early stage, professionals who communicate with them must understand that non-verbal communication is very important. People experiencing dementia are very aware of facial expression and body language. They must not feel as if the person trying to communicate with them is in a hurry, as that leads to stress and has a negative impact on the communication process. Professionals must always introduce themselves by name and title or say what they are going to do, and whenever possible show an item that reinforces what is being communicated.

EXAMPLE

'Hello Mrs. Smith. I am Nancy your nurse today. I am going to take your blood pressure now.' (Show the blood pressure machine/cuff.) 'Is that alright with you?'

In the early stage of dementia, people lose their train of thought and forget what they want to say or have difficulty finding the right words. This is very frustrating. Helping the person to find the word or simply holding their hand, and providing reassurance that you are with them and not to worry, will lower their stress enough that the words will suddenly appear.

Professionals should use short sentences and descriptive words that are easily understood – the fewer medical terms used, the easier the person experiencing dementia will understand what is being said. If possible, use simple pictures or demonstrate what you are saying to reinforce the communication.

I like to use a wipe-off board where I can write 'nurse visits on Thursday'. If the person can remember to cross off the days, a calendar is helpful, especially if he or she needs to take medication. Pill containers have the day on them and the person can connect the date on the calendar with the medication dispenser for taking the correct medication.

People experiencing early stage dementia might also have terminal ill-health such as cancer or heart disease. The person may be receiving palliative care or hospice services because of those medical problems. Professionals must be aware of the person's short-term memory loss, which could result in safety concerns. The person will need everything written down and should be assessed for safety concerns if they are living alone.

MIDDLE STAGE OF DEMENTIA

In the middle stage of the disease, the person may be in an assisted living community (in the UK they are residential care homes) or a nursing home. Medical interventions like hospitalisations may result in more burdens than benefits. The potential for rehabilitation is poor, and someone like George (*see* pp. 173–4) who had reached the stage of memory loss when he could not remember taking his walker even if it were brightly coloured, or could not comprehend what not being weight-bearing on one foot was, would not be a good candidate for surgery for a broken hip. At this stage, medical interventions must be looking at the negative impact of a hospitalisation. When residents in nursing homes or assisted living communities return from a hospital stay, they are often unsteady on their feet, have poor nutritional status and may have a pressure ulcer. Staying in a nursing home where staff know the resident is a palliative approach to the situation when curing is not possible but maintaining function is a reasonable goal.

Behaviour symptoms of dementia and management of the symptoms

In this stage, 'behavioural symptoms' occur. People experiencing moderate dementia may walk around (wander), pace, go into other people's rooms and 'shop' (pick up things) and often with short-term memory loss, they live in another time. Although we are not expecting a cure for AD any time soon, or a medication that will significantly slow the progression of memory loss, we do know how to care for people with memory loss.

When working with professionals and families, I explain that whenever people experiencing memory loss who live in the past are having a problem, they should be creative and 'fix the problem' by agreeing with the reality as the person with memory loss sees it. These are not lies; they are how we help people live experiencing AD.

> **Case Study 11.3 – Ann**
>
> Ann (80) thinks she is living in a hotel. Every morning she goes to the nurses' station and thanks the staff for a wonderful stay. She believes her husband John is coming to pick her up to take her home to care for their small children. The nurses tell Ann how much they have enjoyed having her as a guest and suggest that she have breakfast while waiting for him to arrive. She happily has her breakfast and forgets all about going home until the next morning.

SELF-ASSESSMENT EXERCISE 11.2 (*SEE* ANSWERS ON P. 186)

Time: 20 minutes

- **Trying to get home** – It's 3 o'clock in the afternoon and Shirley feels as if she must go home to be there when her children come home from school. She does not believe that her children are all grown up. How would you 'fix the problem'?
- **Trying to go to work** – Dennis needs to go to work now and is pounding on the door. How would you 'fix the problem'?
- **Refusing to take a shower** – Janet needs to have a shower and she is very resistant to doing this, assuring staff that she has just taken one. You know that she was a very religious person and attended church every Sunday. How would you 'fix the problem'?

Sexuality

Couples may have some problems with remaining sexual, as the person experiencing dementia may not recognise their spouse. Short-term memory has disappeared and the person often lives in the past where they remember their spouse at an early time. I sometimes hear sons quite embarrassed that their mother has been inappropriate sexually with them, thinking that the son is their spouse.

In other cases, especially in nursing homes, married residents will find their 'spouse' (another resident) and with their short-term memory loss, staff cannot convince them that their spouse is living outside of the home. It is heart-breaking for a wife to come for a visit and find her husband holding hands with another resident. Occasionally they are still sexually active, and this causes problems for the families as well as the nursing home staff, who must decide if the two residents are capable of making decisions about their sexual actions.

When professionals begin to see a couple's relationship starting it is justifiable and good practice to call the families to set up a meeting. Usually the nurse or social worker is responsible for setting up the meeting. It is best to have separate meetings with each family to find out how they feel about their loved one becoming a 'couple', and perhaps having a sexual relationship with another resident. If the residents are not married and it appears that they are comfortable and happy with their relationship, the professional continues to monitor them for safety reasons. Resident's rights must be respected and sometimes in the United States the ombudsman assigned to the home is called on to assess the situation. Assisted living communities do not have a social worker or ombudsman, so the nurse in charge, house manager or the executive director is responsible for setting up the meetings.

As with the earlier stage of memory loss, sometimes discussing sexual issues with members of a support group who may have also been confronted with these problems may be helpful. Rarely do I see what is termed 'inappropriate sexual behaviour'. When a person takes off their clothes in front of others, it is usually because they are hot. A man urinating in the potted plant just cannot find the bathroom and a man grabbing at a professional trying to bathe him, may not have received the proper signals that he was going to be showered. When we instruct professionals to bring items to help people who experience memory loss understand what is being asked of them, the 'inappropriate behaviour' disappears. When cueing a person that it is bath time, showing him or her a bar of soap, towel and bathrobe may help her or him to cooperate while taking a shower. If that does not work, and the shower can wait, the professional must leave and try again at another time.

Meaningful activities

At this stage, people experiencing dementia in nursing homes or assisted living communities will rarely if ever engage in meaningful activities. When observing people not engaged in an activity programme I noticed they often fell, wandered into other resident's rooms, sometimes taking others' belongings they thought were theirs, or just fell asleep until the next activity or meal. I developed a concept of 'continuous activities' that began right after breakfast to before lunch, right after lunch or after a nap to before dinner.[8] Activities were then planned until it was time for bed.

The Club

The programme I developed is called 'The Club' and is based on research showing factors lowering the risk of developing a dementia. It has physical and mental exercises, a volunteer programme to help the resident continue to feel needed, and programmes that are just fun. When The Club was part of the culture of the nursing home, scheduled every day, the use of antipsychotics decreased[8] and in one home the number of falls in a month went from 17 to 7 to 5 since The Club was implemented. With the number of falls decreasing so dramatically, the number of hospitalisations also decreased. Families would often not want to hospitalise their loved one as they would miss being in The Club! Quality of life was the goal.

The Club day begins right after breakfast. Some residents eat independently or are early risers and they either stay in the dining room and fall asleep or wander about the neighbourhood. I developed a 'volunteer activity'. In some homes, we have the people who eat independently and are typically looking for something to do while other residents are eating; they eat at the end of the room where we can easily give them projects to do while they are waiting for The Club to start. Volunteer activities may include sorting playing cards, buttons, poker chips or items used for craft projects. In one home staff brought in their 'junk mail' and residents were delighted to open all of the mail and decide in which pile it belonged. Another useful activity is cutting coupons. The professional outlines the coupon so that residents using safe scissors could cut them out and give them to staff. Residents loved feeling that they could help people who worked in their home and the professionals appreciated getting coupons all cut out for them.

When the majority of residents have finished breakfast, everything is put away for the next day and the programme begins with a familiar routine that involves greeting each resident by name and saying something special about him or her. This is followed by an American tradition of saying the Pledge of Allegiance and singing the National Anthem. In the UK, the day begins with the greeting and then talking about the day and what is planned.

We use a wipe-off board for reinforcing what has been said. In the mid-stage of AD, residents do not know the day or often even the month; we do not mention the year as sometimes this is disturbing to residents who are living in the past. This activity might start as follows.

The activity professional

'I never can remember the month, but I do know that last month was September … so this month would be …?' Residents can answer this question and the word is spelled out on the wipe-off board. The 'activity professional' might tell the residents that he or she is a terrible speller, and could someone help her or him spell out October. Each response from the residents is greeted with a 'thank you for being my speller'. We are always trying to find ways to boost the self-esteem of residents. After the month has been written on the board, the activity professional tells the group she or he can never remember the date but he or she does remember that yesterday was the 10th and a resident will respond with 'today is the 11th'. Again, they are thanked and the date is noted on the board. Then the activity professional might say 'let's see if we can name 11 words that remind us of the fall' (autumn). That is a right-brain activity. After six words have been offered, the activity professional will do the math on the board: 'we need 11 and let's count how many we have [counting], then 5 from 11 is …?' This is a left-brain activity.

This activity is followed by a discussion of the day's news that may be from the *Daily Chronicle* US (see www.activityconnection.com), and the *Daily Sparkle* UK (see www.dailysparkle.co.uk/info-pack-landing). I hesitate to use the newspaper, as it is full of not so happy news.

The day continues with a schedule of activities that are planned to meet the individual interests of residents, will stimulate them physically and keep their brain active. Table 11.1 offers a sample of a typical day.

TABLE 11.1 The Club activities

Volunteers at work	Afternoon delight
Meet and Greet	Fun and Games
News and Views	Afternoon Tea and Chat
Exercise	Brain Games
Second Cup	Food Trivia
Morning Surprise	Dance to Dine
Food Trivia	Word Games
Dance to Dine	Movie Classic

Spirituality

Weekends include spiritual/religious programmes representing the various faiths of residents attending The Club. In the middle stage of dementing ill-health, many residents can still say a prayer and take communion. Clergy must be aware that some residents may have trouble swallowing, so whenever possible a professional should be with them during communion.

Sundays are planned so that families, especially the grandchildren, can have fun with a person who has memory loss and may not remember their name.

KEY POINT 11.5

It is essential for families to understand how important it is to keep connected as a family, and that in spite of memory loss the person experiencing dementia can sense love and can still enjoy a dish or cone of ice cream!

Communication

It is important to remember that the person's short-term and moderate-term memory is damaged in the middle stage of dementing ill-health. Writing things down is usually not effective. However, showing the person items to help give clues about what is being communicated continues to be helpful. Pantomiming using gestures may also help a person experiencing dementia understand what is being said or asked of them. Many times, a man is viewed as being sexually inappropriate when he grabs a woman undressing him for a shower. Showing him a towel, soap and bathrobe and making gestures of taking a shower may help him understand the need for undressing.

It may be difficult for people to express pain in words, so careful watching of non-verbal messages, as well as sounds, can help assess pain (*see* Chapter 8). The PAINAD (see www.healthcare.uiowa.edu/igec/tools/pain/PAINAD.pdf) is one tool that professionals can use to assess pain in people with moderate and advanced dementia.[9]

LATE STAGE

A year after the first 'club' was implemented I received a call from the administrator asking me to come back and develop a special programme for residents who were in the last stage of AD and could no longer participate in The Club programmes. This was also the time when families were counselled that a palliative approach to care was in the best interests of the residents, when comfort was the goal. That meant no cardio-pulmonary resuscitation (CPR), hospitalisation, tube feeding or treating generalised infections with antibiotics.[10]

SELF-ASSESSMENT EXERCISE 11.3

> **Time: 10 minutes**
> How would you initiate a conversation about end-of-life care for people experiencing advanced AD and the futility of medical interventions at this time of life?

The administrator felt that we needed to have a special programme like The Club to show families that the staff were not just keeping residents experiencing advanced dementia groomed, fed, changed and put in front of a television programme they could not understand, or 'parked' in front of the nurses' station so they could be watched and become invisible.

Namaste Care™

> ### KEY POINT 11.6
> Namaste Care™ is a palliative care approach meaning to 'honour the spirit within'.

Meaningful activities for people experiencing advanced dementia needed to be sensory with a 'loving touch' approach to programming. The result was Namaste Care™, a programme that has grown from one nursing home to hundreds of nursing homes, assisted living communities and hospice organisations in the United States, Australia and the United Kingdom.[11] Namaste is a Hindu word that has many meanings, but the one I saw when I was searching for this programme's name is 'to honour the spirit within'. Every aspect of Namaste Care™ honours the resident from the moment they are taken to the room where the programme is taking place until they leave for lunch or dinner.

The Namaste Care™ room has been prepared before the residents arrive to help them feel a sense of peace when they are taken into the room. Lights are lowered; the scent of lavender permeates the air as there is some evidence that this scent may lower anxiety and disruptive behaviour.[12] Soothing music is playing and the room or space is made to look as homelike as possible.

Namaste Care™ is a seven-day-a-week programme just like The Club and it takes place at least four hours a day. Namaste Care™ is person-centred and 'honouring the spirit within' begins when the resident enters the Namaste Care™ room and is greeted by the staff called 'Namaste Carers', in a manner that is comfortable and meaningful for the resident. Dr Collins has his hand shaken, Aunt Dottie is hugged and Marge is told how beautiful she always looks. Each resident is helped into a reclining chair, if they do not arrive in one, as a wheelchair is not comfortable for people experiencing advanced dementia. A blanket is tucked around the person and a beverage is offered.

Continuous hydration is a major activity in the Namaste Care™ day. A cup with the person's name on it is close to them so that there is no confusion as to where their beverage is and it is convenient for families as well as the professional to offer a beverage throughout the Namaste Care™ day. It is difficult to keep a person experiencing advanced dementia hydrated and the result may be urinary tract infections and skin tears. Urinary tract infections account for many hospitalisations.[13] Professionals in nursing/care homes and assisted living communities report that people experiencing advanced dementia who are hospitalised often return malnourished, sometimes with a catheter, or more medication than when they were in their care and with loss of function. A variety of juices and flavoured water are always available so residents have choice. A list of all residents in the programme who have swallowing difficulties or have special dietary needs is located in the Namaste Care™ room and is kept current.

In addition, the Namaste Care™ room is stocked with puddings, ice cream and ingredients for 'smoothies' and other food items that the individual enjoys eating. A meaningful activity for one resident was to have several Fig Newtons, cookies he remembered enjoying when he was a young boy. One of the consequences of advanced AD is weight loss, therefore the added calories and increased intake of beverages is beneficial from a medical perspective as well as an enjoyable activity for the residents.

When the majority of residents attending Namaste Care™ are in the room they are assessed for pain or discomfort using the PAINAD scale[9] and professionals are notified if there are any concerns that the person is not comfortable.

KEY POINT 11.7

Quality of life is not possible if a person is uncomfortable.

Then a basin of warm water is taken to the person and activities of daily living (ADLs – see http://en.wikipedia.org/wiki/Activities_of_daily_living for more information) are offered in an unhurried way. The foundation of Namaste Care™ is 'the power of loving touch', and with this approach to care small miracles occur.[14] Faces are gently washed and moisturised with a face cream that has a scent from the past. In the United States, the most popular moisturiser for women was Ponds Cold Cream and the aftershave for men was Old Spice. As part of the person-centred approach to care, families are asked if their loved one used any particular moisturisers or aftershave and the families provide the items, or the community purchases them.

The person's hands are washed or soaked in a basin of warm water, and hands and arms are moisturised. One of the most enjoyable activities seems to be having their hair combed or scalp massaged. This may remind the person of when their mother combed their hair. While offering these activities, the professional talks to the person in a soft, soothing way. Those people who are non-verbal will often spontaneously respond by saying, 'thank you' or 'I love you' to the professional or their families.[15]

Some people enjoy having a lifelike dog or cat to hold, others find comfort with realistic looking babies. One resident's life was changed when she found her baby. She had been a resident who stayed in her room most of the time. There was no family to provide information about her and staff assumed that she had been a 'loner' most of her adult life. She rarely attended activities and even more rarely smiled. She wandered into the Namaste Care™ room, spotted this realistic-looking doll and took her gently in her arms and said: 'At last I've found you. I've been looking for you my whole life'! Now that she has her 'baby' and believes the baby wants to go to activities, she and her 'baby' are very busy and when this person is told by staff what a wonderful mother she is, she now smiles most of the time.[16]

Before lunch, residents need to be stimulated, so they will be awake for their meals. Music from the big band era or Broadway musicals is played. Lights are turned up and something fun like bubbles and sensory items from the season or holidays are shown to residents, who like to hold them and may talk about what memories they help recall. This often produces happy smiles and comments. In the fall (autumn), small gourds or pumpkins and the scent of cinnamon may jog memories of this season. One winter, staff brought a tub of snow to the Namaste Care™ room and the residents tried to make snowballs! Residents are taken to the toilet, and prepared for their meal. Each resident is thanked for coming to Namaste Care™ and most are hugged as they leave the room.

After lunch, if the residents do not have to go to bed because of a skin problem, e.g. an existing or potential pressure ulcer, they return to the Namaste Care™ room for the afternoon activities. These include foot soaking and moisturising, a range of motion to music, hand massages and back rubs, or anything that the professional believes is an enjoyable and meaningful activity.

Families often visit in the afternoon and they are invited to participate in the programme. Some families report that the visits are longer and more meaningful to the family member who has had difficulty visiting their loved one who does not remember them and is non-verbal.[17] Richard Taylor experiences dementia, and has eloquently written about his feelings about his future:

> I want and need to give and receive love. Even when I can't remember your name, will you please love me?[18]

KEY POINT 11.8

Families who have selected medical interventions, even when their love one is in the advanced stage, who feel as if they have to do something, are comforted by the palliative care approach offered in Namaste Care™.

Case Study 11.4 – Bill

Bill visited his mother twice every day. She was in the advanced stage of dementia and was not hungry or thirsty. Bill had recently retired and was divorced; all he had to focus on was his mother. I would see him pleading for her to take one more bite, one more sip, but most of the time she would not. On the day we opened Namaste Care™, I found his mother sitting in a wheelchair in front of the nurses' station. Her frail little arms were black and blue. She had stopped drinking and her son ordered his mother to be taken to the hospital for intravenous hydration. We took her to the Namaste Care™ room, settled her in a lounge chair, tucked a quilt around her and gave her a lollipop to suck on. When Bill could not find his mother he panicked, but was told she had been taken to a new programme. Bill stood at the door, looked at his mother and burst into tears. I went over to him and asked what was wrong. He said that his mother looked so happy he was overcome with emotion. When Bill heard that this programme would take place every day he went to the nurses and told them he never wanted his mother hospitalised again.

This is just one example of how Namaste Care™ shows how a palliative approach to care is not just about 'not doing something' but is about 'doing what is appropriate and meaningful' for people in the advanced stage of AD. While the programme began for people experiencing advanced dementia, it has enhanced the lives of people with a variety of diseases, who benefit from the loving touch approach to care.

The results from the Namaste Care™ programme include a decrease in the use of anti-psychotics and anti-anxiety medication, and lowered incidence of behavioural symptoms of dementia, especially resistance to care and agitation. In several studies, families and professionals report increased satisfaction with Namaste Care™.[19] This programme can be implemented without adding staff, or a separate room dedicated to the programme, and supplies are not costly.

CONCLUSIONS

KEY POINT 11.9

A palliative care approach is appropriate for all stages of Alzheimer's disease.

The goals of care change as disease progresses. For instance, hospitalisation and even surgery may be appropriate for someone in the early stage of an irreversible dementia, but by the middle and last stages, hospitalisation and most medical interventions have more burdens associated with them than any benefits. The person with early stage dementia might also have another more critical terminal ill-health problem.

We do not have either a cure for AD on the horizon, or medication that will significantly slow the progression of memory loss, but what we do have are approaches that can help a person live and not just exist with significant memory loss. Dame Cicely

Saunders the founder of the modern hospice movement, spoke of the hospice goal as:

> not only to help you die peacefully, but also to live until you die (see www.
> lifebeforedeath.com/thelastword/deathquotes.shtml).

Involving the person experiencing dementia in meaningful activities, joining their journey rather than trying to pull them into a world they no longer understand, helps professional caregivers and families feel less helpless. The need for simple touch is reciprocal throughout the course of dementia and brings smiles from both the person with memory loss and their caregivers, both professional and family.[17]

> **KEY POINT 11.10**
>
> The power of loving touch is not to be underestimated. It is the foundation of how we truly care for people experiencing dementia.

ACKNOWLEDGEMENT

A special thanks to my husband Ladislav Volicer for his help with the references and advice on this chapter.

REFERENCES

1 Myers B. Alzheimer's cost expected to balloon 500 percent by 2050. *Provider.* 2013; **39**: 10.
2 Gillick M, Berkman S, Cullen L. A patient-centered approach to advance medical planning in the nursing home. *Journal of the American Geriatric Society.* 1999; **47**: 227–30.
3 Saliba D, Kington R, Buchanan J, *et al.* Appropriateness of the decision to transfer nursing facility residents to the hospital. *Journal of the American Geriatric Society.* 2000; **48**: 154–63.
4 Volpato S, Onder G, Cavalieri M, *et al.* Characteristics of nondisabled older patients developing new disability associated with medical illnesses and hospitalization. *Journal of General Internal Medicine.* 2007; **22**: 668–74.
5 Abdelmalek C, Goyal S, Narula A, *et al.* Advance directives: give teeth to end-of-life choices. *Aging Well.* 2013; **6**: 25–7.
6 Gray BH. England's approach to improving end-of-life care: a strategy for honoring patients' choices. *Issue Brief (Commonwealth Fund).* 2011; **15**(July): 1–15.
7 Larson EB, Shadlen MF, Wang L, *et al.* Survival after initial diagnosis of Alzheimer disease. *Annals of Internal Medicine.* 2004; **140**: 501–9.
8 Volicer L, Simard J, Pupa JH, *et al.* Effects of continuous activity programming on behavioral symptoms of dementia. *Journal of the American Medical Directors Association.* 2006; **7**: 426–31.
9 Warden V, Hurley AC, Volicer L. Development and psychometric evaluation of the PAINAD (Pain Assessment in Advanced Dementia) Scale. *Journal of the American Medial Directors Association.* 2003; **4**: 9–15.
10 Volicer L. Hospice and palliative care. In: Agronin ME, Maletta GJ, editors. *Principles and Practice of Geriatric Psychiatry.* 2nd ed. Philadelphia: Lippincott Williams & Wilkins; 2011. pp. 235–45.
11 Simard J. *The End-of-Life Namaste Program for People with Dementia.* 2nd ed. Baltimore/London/Sydney: Health Professions Press; 2013.
12 Fu CY, Moyle W, Cooke M. A randomised controlled trial of the use of aromatherapy and hand massage to reduce disruptive behaviour in people with dementia. *BMC Complementary and Alternative Medicine.* 2013; **13**: 165.

13 Sampson EL, Blanchard MR, Jones L, *et al*. Dementia in the acute hospital: prospective cohort study of prevalence and mortality. *British Journal of Psychiatry*. 2009; **195**: 61–6.

14 Simard J. One small miracle. *Journal of Gerontological Nursing*. 2012; **38**: 52–6.

15 Simard J. Three simple words. *Australian Journal of Dementia Care*. 2013; **1**: 21.

16 Simard J. At last I found you. *Gerontological Nursing*. 2013; **39**: 55–6.

17 Nicholls D, Chang E, Johnson A, *et al*. Touch, the essence of caring for people with end-stage dementia: a mental health perspective in Namaste Care. *Aging & Mental Health*. 2013; **17**: 571–8.

18 Taylor R. *Alzheimer's from the Inside Out*. Baltimore, MD: Health Professions Press; 2007.

19 Stacpoole M, Wen A. *Personal Communication*. 2013.

TO LEARN MORE

- www.namastecare.com (accessed 11 March 2014)
- www.alz.org (accessed 11 March 2014)
- www.alzheimers.org.uk (accessed 11 March 2014)
- Simard J. *The End-of-Life Namaste Program for People with Dementia*. 2nd ed. Baltimore/London/Sydney: Health Professions Press; 2013.
- Volicer L, Simard J. Management of advanced dementia. In: Weiner MF, Lipton AM, editors. *Textbook of Alzheimer Disease and Other Dementias*. Arlington, VA: American Psychiatric Publishing. 2009; pp. 333–49.
- Stettinius M. *Inside the Dementia Epidemic*. Horsehead, NY: Dundee-Lakemont Press; 2012.

ANSWERS TO SELF-ASSESSMENT EXERCISE 11.1 (*SEE* P. 175)

- **Driving** – David's wife tells him that his licence is lost and he cannot drive without it. Until they can make an appointment to get another, she will drive but needs him to be the navigator. He can hold the GPS or she can print out directions that he can read for her. If he cannot read, he can hold the map for her just in case she needs to look at it.
- **Dressing** – Sara's outfits are laid out on a chair near her bed so that she can easily see what she has selected. If she does not put on an appropriate outfit, she is told that this Sunday is a dress-up day or casual day – the opposite of what she is wearing.
- **Playing cards** – The women who play bridge with Aileen let her know that they have decided to disband for the month, or for the summer. When they visit, a simple card game is suggested. The rules are 'bent' for Aileen so that she wins most of the time.

ANSWERS TO SELF-ASSESSMENT EXERCISE 11.2 (*SEE* P. 177)

- **Trying to get home** – Staff reassure Shirley that the children are with grandmother or are at a friend's house playing.
- **Trying to go to work** – Dennis is reminded that this is the weekend or that he is on vacation.
- **Refusing to take a shower** – Janet is told that this is Saturday night and she needs to take a bath to be ready to dress up for church the next day.

CHAPTER 12

Creutzfeldt–Jakob disease and palliative care

Kay de Vries

INTRODUCTION

This chapter discusses palliative care for people experiencing Creutzfeldt–Jakob disease (CJD) and their families. A background to CJD is presented along with a discussion on diagnosis, disease trajectory and the experiences of the person with CJD at the end-of-life. The chapter also addresses the risk of contamination from CJD, issues and challenges related to stigma, genetic testing and counselling, bereavement and loss, and advance care planning.

CREUTZFELDT–JAKOB DISEASE (CJD)

CJD is a rare and fatal neurodegenerative disease first described in the 1920s. It has historically been classified within the dementia syndromes because the symptoms that occur over the disease progression contain all of those that are experienced in other dementia syndromes, but at an accelerated pace. It is recognised as both a dementia syndrome and an acute neurological illness. CJD belongs to a group of diseases known as transmissible spongiform encephalopathies (TSE) that are known to occur in both humans and animals. The progress of multifocal encephalopathies is aggressive and brain damage that occurs is characterised by the spongy appearance of brain tissue seen under a microscope. It is also referred to as prion disease, an acronym for a proteinaceous infectious agent. The prion theory suggests that the infective agent of CJD is only composed of protein and does not contain nucleic acid, which would be necessary if the agent was a conventional virus. The transmittable agent is either genetic or an abnormal form of prion protein that causes aggregates of cellular protein to accumulate in the brain. The exact process that occurs that leads to brain damage from original inoculation/contamination is incompletely understood.[1,2,3,4]

Four types of CJD have been identified:

1 iatrogenic
2 inherited
3 sporadic
4 variant CJD.

Iatrogenic CJD refers to the cases of CJD that have been caused by medical treatment. These comprise a very small number of cases. The causes include:

➤ injections of infected human-derived growth hormone (hGH) and human gonadotrophin (hGN)
➤ tissue grafts, particularly corneal transplants and human dura mater grafts
➤ contamination from neurosurgical instruments and depth electrodes.[2,5,6]

More recently iatrogenic CJD has occurred as a result of a CJD-contaminated blood transfusion.[7,8,9]

Inherited CJD occurs where there is a mutation in the prion protein gene that makes conversion into the abnormal form more likely. Approximately 10% of the cases of CJD are inherited and the most common of these are Gerstmann–Sträussler–Scheinker Syndrome (GSS), Fatal Familial Insomnia (FFI) and familial CJD, and account for 7–15% of all cases of CJD.[2,10,11] Sporadic CJD (also referred to as classical CJD) refers to cases of CJD that occur at random throughout the world. They are categorised as sporadic if they have no genetic mutation or any known iatrogenic infection. Sporadic CJD accounts for 85% of all cases of CJD and has a median age at death of 65 years.[6] In 1996, in the United Kingdom (UK), a new variant of CJD was officially recognised[12,13] and is believed to be linked to the bovine spongiform encephalopathy (BSE) outbreak during the 1980s.[14,15] It is widely accepted that the BSE epidemic that occurred in the mid-1980s originated from animals consuming feed that was contaminated with scrapie, a sheep prion disease.

Other more rare types of spongiform encephalopathies include 'kuru'. Kuru is a TSE that was confined to the Fore social group or tribe, and amongst other groups who intermarried with the Fore group, in the Eastern highlands of Papua New Guinea. It was transmitted through an endocannibalistic ritual associated with mourning. Women and children comprised the majority of kuru victims.[16,17] Kuru is now very rarely found amongst this group due to the cessation of cannibalism in Papua New Guinea.[17]

KEY POINT 12.1

CJD is a rare and fatal neurodegenerative disease also known as prion disease. There are four recognised types:
1 **iatrogenic** – refers to the cases of CJD that have been caused by medical treatment
2 **inherited** – occurs where there is a mutation in the prion protein gene
3 **sporadic** – (classical CJD) are cases of CJD that occur at random
4 **variant CJD** – believed to be linked to the BSE outbreak during the 1980s.

DIAGNOSIS OF CJD

CJD is always fatal, is very difficult to diagnose and is unique in that it is both genetic and transmissible. Early diagnosis is an important aspect in relation to the management of the disease. Diagnosis of all forms of CJD is made by clinical and neuropathological examination and conclusive diagnosis can only be made by microscopic examination of brain tissue.[13,18] Investigations include electroencephalogram (EEG), magnetic resonance imaging (MRI) and lumbar puncture, where 14-3-3 brain protein in cerebral spinal fluid (CSF) has been identified as a marker for transmissible spongiform encephalopathies.[19] The number of confirmed cases of CJD has risen steadily in recent years. It is believed that this may be due to more accurate diagnosis and an increased awareness of the disease, but also due to the emergence of variant CJD.[6]

RISK OF CONTAMINATION/INFECTION FROM CJD

To date, four cases of CJD in the UK have been identified through blood transfusion transmission.[8,15] These people received blood in 1999 or earlier from donors who were later diagnosed with variant CJD.[20] Some tissues pose a greater risk of infection than others and the highest risk is from contact with the brain (including dura mater), spinal cord and eye tissue.[9] Common challenges within studies on contamination and CJD include access to and content of past medical/dental treatment records for diseases with long incubation periods.[2,21] As Ludlam and Turner[11] point out, management of the risk of transmission of prion diseases by blood and plasma products remains highly problematic. Despite the falling number of clinical cases in the UK, up to 90% of infected persons may sustain long-term preclinical or subclinical disease and these are in the 20–40 years age group, which would suggest that there is a significant pool of potentially infectious blood donors.[11] Therefore further research and continuing surveillance is required to assess the risk of transmission between individuals. More recently a prototype blood test for diagnosis of CJD in symptomatic people has been developed, which in the future could allow development of large-scale screening tests for asymptomatic variant CJD.[22] The risk of CJD transmission from the individual to professionals is minimal. However, normal precautions should be maintained when dealing with human body tissue.[23]

REFLECTIVE PRACTICE EXERCISE 12.1

Time: 20 minutes
- Consider how you would support a person who was undergoing investigations to determine whether they had CJD following an event of contamination as a result of a medical procedure.
- Reflect on how the type of conversation you would engage in and what your position would be in relation to disclosing the information to the person.
- Think about the process of breaking bad news. What would be your position in regard to this?
- Consider breaking bad news principles; 'endorsing' bad news; 'picking up the pieces'; supporting medical clinician availability; and information giving.

CLINICAL PROGRESS OF CJD

There is no cure for CJD and the clinical presentation, progressive nature of the disease and failure to find any other diagnosis are the hallmarks of the disease. CJD is characterised by a rapidly progressive dementia (of less than two years), together with at least two of the following symptoms:

➤ myoclonus (muscle twitches or spasms and involuntary jerky type movements)
➤ visual or cerebellar problems
➤ extrapyramidal or pyramidal signs
➤ akinetic mutism.[2,6]

Initial signs of ill-health may be non-specific with complaints of.
➤ dizziness
➤ sleep disturbances
➤ mood swings

➤ headache
➤ apathy
➤ depression.

Neurological symptoms for sporadic and variant CJD develop and progress extremely quickly. Cognitive processes, such as memory, concentration and problem-solving, are affected and the person may become disoriented. Movement is affected, particularly balance and gait, and the person may become apraxic (unable to perform complex sequential tasks) and experience a tremor and rigidity. Ataxia (not to be confused with apraxia) is a common neurological sign and consists of lack of voluntary co-ordination of muscle movements.[24]

Speech becomes slurred and quiet (dysarthria), the person will have word-finding difficulties as the content of language is reduced and reading and writing deteriorates. As the ill-health progresses, swallowing difficulties and visual disturbances occur and at later stages there may be cortical blindness. The person may experience seizures in the final stages. A distinguishing feature of variant CJD is the presence of persistent painful sensory symptoms such as paraesthesia (pins and needles) and/or dysaesthesia (pain arising or persisting from innocuous touch).[10,25]

Iatrogenic CJD has a slightly different clinical progress where dementia is not a prominent feature.[6] The incubation period for iatrogenic CJD ranges from 5 to 42 years (mean 17 years) and, unlike sporadic CJD, signs and symptoms almost never include dementia. If dementia symptoms do occur, this is typically at an advanced stage of the clinical course. According to Brown *et al.*,[26] the era of iatrogenic CJD is nearly over, with only occasional cases that have had exceptionally long incubation periods still being diagnosed.

Variant CJD is also distinguished from other types of CJD by the:
➤ age of onset
➤ duration of symptoms
➤ mode of occurrence.

➤ symptom profile
➤ histopathology

The median duration of ill-health from onset of first symptoms to death is 13 months (range 6–36 months) for variant CJD, compared to a disease trajectory of four months (range 1–74 months) for sporadic CJD.[8,10] The average age of onset of variant CJD is

28 years (compared to 65 years for the median age at death for sporadic CJD), with a range of 12–74 years reported.[6,13] However, based on one case of variant CJD diagnosed in a 74-year-old, some concerns have been expressed that variant CJD may be misdiagnosed as Alzheimer's disease in the older population.[19,27,28]

During the early stages of ill-health, people experiencing CJD usually experience mental health symptoms; this is a particular manifestation of variant CJD.[8,25,29,30] These symptoms most commonly take the form of depression or, less often, a schizophrenia-like psychosis. A misdiagnosis may mean that the person is treated inappropriately with antidepressant or antipsychotic medications and people experiencing CJD may be referred to mental health services in the early stages of the ill-health.[30,31,32,33] Referral to mental health services has been found to cause distress to family members, particularly if the person died while still in a mental health unit.[29]

REFLECTIVE PRACTICE EXERCISE 12.2

Time: 5 minutes
- Consider how the individual may feel about a diagnosis of CJD.
- How might you prepare people for and support them during and after the investigations?

KEY POINT 12.2

There is no cure for CJD. The neurological symptoms experienced by the person with CJD near the end-of-life can be extremely distressing, both for the individual and for their caregivers. It is important that families and caregivers are prepared for this.

MANAGEMENT OF SYMPTOMS OF CJD

KEY POINT 12.3

There is no cure for CJD and palliation is the only treatment.

Once the ill-health is diagnosed, people experiencing CJD may be cared for in a variety of settings. These include:
- general hospital wards
- neurological units
- hospices
- care homes
- the person's own or family homes.

Due to the complexity of the physical symptoms, input from professionals with palliative care expertise is an important consideration.[31,33,34,35] People experiencing CJD experience a myriad of symptoms as outlined above. The control of these is complex and requires careful assessment and expertise in symptom management (*see* Table 12.1).

TABLE 12.1 Common symptoms and methods of management

Symptom	Management
Myoclonus	• Minimal movement when touching, turning or repositioning the person • Maintaining a quiet environment • Levetiracetam, valporate sodium and benzodiazepines such as clonazepam
Spasticity	• Baclofen, dantrolene and diazepam, although these are less effective in the presence of muscle rigidity
Ataxia	• This is extremely difficult to treat and there are in most cases no effective medications
Visual hallucinations	• Respond well to drugs used in Alzheimer's disease, e.g. donepezil, galantamine and rivastigmine
Aggression and agitation	• Atypical antipsychotic drugs such as quetiapine, risperidone or olanzapine • Diazepam can also sometimes help
Pain	• Assessment of pain is difficult due to communication problems • Potential for pain exists in the presence of spasticity, hypereflexia, mouth infections and bladder and bowel disturbance • The Analgesic Ladder should be used in assessing and managing pain (*see* Figure 12.1)[36]
Paraesthesia and/or dysaesthesia	• Gabapentin, pregabalin and amitriptyline are all useful for neuropathic pain of this type
Heightened startle reflex	• Non-pharmacological approaches such as: communicating calmly and gently; using minimal and gentle touch; ensuring minimal sound; playing soft familiar music; using soft lighting
Swallowing difficulties (dysphagia)	• Thickened fluids and puréed food • Appropriate positioning to reduce the risk of aspiration • Any decision to institute measures such as naso-gastric tube feeding or nutrition via a gastrostomy need to be carefully considered and negotiated with family
Increased salivation as result of swallowing difficulties	• Can be managed by drugs that reduce the amount of saliva such as atropine drops or hyoscine patches
Mouth infections, e.g. candida albicans	• Mouth care is important in relation to preventing infection and maintaining comfort • May be difficult to carry out in the presence of myoclonic jerking • Administration of analgesia such as paracetamol may help facilitate mouth care
Urinary frequency	• Urinary antispasmodics such as tolterodine
Urinary incontinence	• Frequent, scheduled toileting • Incontinent pads • If skin breakdown is of concern or the end-of-life is approaching, urinary catheterisation will reduce the need for frequent touching and turning when changing continence pads or wet beds
Constipation	• Occurs as a result of reduced fluid intake, immobility and the effects of neurological disturbance on the bowel • Careful balance is required in the management of this between over-intervention and distress from unrelieved constipation

Adapted from: de Vries (2003);[31] Barnett (2002);[34] Barnett & McLean (2005);[10] Prout (2000);[35] Bailey *et al.* (2000);[33] CJD Surveillance Unit (2012).[6]

The World Health Organization (WHO) analgesic ladder (1986)[36] (Figure 12.1) provides a framework for managing pain in palliative care that has good applicability to managing pain in people with CJD.

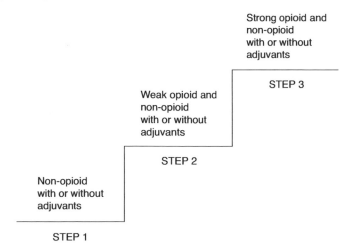

Figure 12.1

The principles within the framework are that the most appropriate analgesic is administered at a dose that relieves pain without causing unmanageable side effects (*see* Table 12.2), combined with the administration of appropriate adjuvants (co-analgesics – *see* Table 12.3; *see* Chapter 8, *Pain Management*).

TABLE 12.2 Principles for the correct use of analgesics

1 The oral form of medication should be favoured whenever possible.

2 Analgesics should be given at regular intervals.

3 The dosage of medication should be adjusted until the person is comfortable.

4 Prescribe the dosage to be taken at definite intervals in accordance with the person's level of pain.

5 Prescribe in accordance to pain intensity as evaluated by a scale of intensity of pain.

6 Dosing of pain medication should be adapted to the person (the correct dosage is one that will allow adequate relief of pain).

7 Regularity of analgesic administration is crucial for the adequate treatment of pain.

8 Analgesics should be prescribed with a constant concern for detail.

Source: Adapted from Vargas-Schaffer (2010)[37]

Adjuvant analgesics are drugs that do not function primarily as analgesics to relieve pain but can act to relieve pain in specific circumstances. For people experiencing CJD the 'usual' list of adjuvants needs to be extended to include therapeutic interventions that have been shown to be beneficial in dementia care practice, such as music therapy, distraction, aromatherapy, and minimising sensory stimulation.[38]

TABLE 12.3 Adjuvant analgesics

Medications	Physical interventions
Non-steroidal anti-inflammatory drugs (NSAIDs)	Transcutaneous electrical nerve stimulation (TENS)
Anticonvulsants	Acupuncture
Muscle relaxants	Chiropractic
Antidepressants	Physiotherapy and physical therapy
Steroids	Local anaesthetics
Antispasmodics	Surgical and neurosurgical procedures
Antibiotics	
Compounds that act synergistically with opioids such as cannabinoids (e.g. nabilone)	

Sources: Adapted from: Vargas-Schaffer (2010);[37] Leung (2012)[39]

KEY POINT 12.4

The complexity of the symptoms experienced by people experiencing CJD at the end-of-life necessitates consultation with experts in palliative care.

CAREGIVING ISSUES

The emergence of variant CJD set in place unprecedented levels of care services for caregivers of people with all types of CJD. In the UK care is now substantially funded and supported and many family members are closely involved with CJD support groups. CJD care is co-ordinated by the team based with the CJD Surveillance Unit in Edinburgh. The team acts as a source of specialist advice regarding care issues and symptom management and support for funding of comprehensive care packages. This is a inter-disciplinary team and includes:

➤ the person's GP and district nurse
➤ palliative care specialists
➤ speech and language therapist
➤ social worker
➤ occupational therapist
➤ a neurologist
➤ physiotherapist
➤ care agency representative
➤ dietician
➤ other relevant personnel.[10]

The uniqueness of CJD, in that it can be both genetic and transmissible, can cause difficulties for family members and caregivers. They may be faced with a range of issues, such as:

➤ general lack of information and awareness at a clinical level
➤ delays in diagnosis
➤ insensitive information provision and breaking bad news by professionals
➤ insensitive approaches by professionals regarding autopsy procedures
➤ delays in autopsy results

> delays in genetic testing
> delayed access to appropriate healthcare services.

STIGMA
REFLECTIVE PRACTICE EXERCISE 12.3

Time: 10 minutes
- Spend time to reflect on stigma and the impact this has on the individual and family.
- If possible, draw on your own experiences of stigma or those of someone you know, and how you or the other person dealt with stigma.
- Make a list of the 'golden rules of caring' that might help you in your personal and professional role.

Stigma has been identified as a significant issue for people experiencing dementia, their families and caregivers. In the case of CJD this was particularly significant if there had been a referral to mental health services in the early stages of the ill-health.[29,30,31,33] Stigma related to mental health symptoms is well described in the literature. CJD is, however, a neurological disorder and common neurological diseases such as Parkinson's disease and epilepsy affect people of all ages and are stigmatising, unpredictable and disabling illnesses.[40] However, little is written on the subject of stigma in relation to many neurological disorders, including CJD.

Stigma for people experiencing CJD may arise on a number of accounts. These can be associated with diagnostic labels that may be applied to neuropsychiatric illness in general[41] and are related to the overt symptoms of CJD, particularly the earlier psychiatric manifestations. Although the age range of people experiencing CJD excludes them from the discussion on stigma, that reflects negative stereotypes of ageing or the aged, it can arise in relation to the symptoms of dementia that occur as the disease progresses. These disease manifestations include changes in outward appearance and competence. The clinical progress of CJD leads to a state of profound dementia and to death, and dementia is a term that has been found to provoke fear and dread in the public.[42,43]

BEREAVEMENT AND LOSS
Bereavement experiences and responses are highly influenced by the manner in which people come to know of their ill-health and how the time was spent between diagnosis and death. Family members and caregivers can experience despair at not being able to keep their promise for a home death, and this has been found to lead to complicated bereavement as they may have made the promise with poor understanding of what to expect as the disease progresses (*see* Chapter 6).[44]

Some of the common challenges faced by families and caregivers of people with late-stage dementia are:
> guilt associated with the institutionalisation of the family member
> lack of familiarity with death in general and death due to advancing dementia

➤ limited understanding of the natural cause of late-stage dementia.[45,46]

KEY POINT 12.5

The opportunity for family and friends to be able to spend quality time with their terminally ill relative and to be able to say their goodbyes has a significant impact on their ability to cope with the loss when it does occur.[44]

Some of the most difficult decisions that families and caregivers are expected to make are about medical care for the person experiencing CJD,[47] and they can experience emotional distress when expected to make decisions about medical treatment on behalf of the person.[48] Family members and caregivers are often unfamiliar with setting goals and making decisions on behalf of another and experience confusion about what actions, or inactions, might impact on the death of their relative (*see* Chapter 5).[45,46] Furthermore, family members may believe that the person experiencing CJD does not have a quality of life and that their misery is prolonged as long as they stay alive[45] (*see* Chapter 13). This is complicated by the variable and unpredictable disease trajectory for CJD, i.e. the period from diagnosis to death may be very short (one month) or prolonged over a number of years, with no means of prognostication of time of death.

Anticipatory grief has been widely studied among family caregivers of people experiencing dementia.[49] This is the process of experiencing bereavement prior to the death and is related to actual and anticipated loss of the personhood and of the relationship shared with the dying person[50] (*see* 'To Learn More', p. 201). It involves multiple losses for family and caregivers (companionship, personal freedom and control) and the person experiencing dementia.[49] Family members of people experiencing dementia often feel that they have lost the person many months and even years before the death. Witnessing cognitive and physical deterioration over a prolonged period of time has been shown to lead to depression, strain and burden.[51] Being a spouse carer and being depressed are the strongest predictors of complicated and normal grief after death.[49]

Inability to communicate can be particularly frustrating, distressing and isolating for the person with CJD, their family members and caregivers.

KEY POINT 12.6

It is important not to assume that people experiencing CJD lack awareness of others and of their environment as there is good evidence that varying levels of awareness are present until a very advanced stage of the ill-health.[52]

The person may also display attachment behaviour as a 'normal' response to extreme distress, ill-health and loss. In the presence of cognitive impairment the inability to adequately express emotions reduces interactions to more 'primitive' responses.[52] In these circumstances it is important that professionals support communication between families and the person experiencing CJD and use alternative methods of communication as they may still enjoy hearing the voices of those they are close to.

GENETIC TESTING FOR CJD

In the case of CJD, families will be faced with both dealing with the impact of the potential or actual loss of the person, as well as possibly facing the prospect of making a decision to have genetic counselling. The proliferation of genetic disorders has led to an increase in referrals to genetic counselling clinics.[53,54,55] The likelihood that a number of prion diseases have a genetic link now means that families of these individuals are being referred to specialist genetic clinics for genetic counselling.[56] The aim of genetic counselling is to:

➤ help and support the individuals and families to understand the genetic condition
➤ appreciate the risk of recurrence
➤ understand the options available
➤ make decisions and adjustments appropriate to their personal and family situation.[54]

However, the majority of people offered testing for CJD choose not to be tested (*see* 'To Learn More', p. 201 – CJD Support Group Network).

It has been suggested that new genetics has medicalised individuals and family members, as well as relationships within families, and has created ethical and practical dilemmas that impact on the person, families and also on medicine as a whole[57,58] (*see* Chapter 3). This medicalised focus can have a profound impact on relationships. Seminal research by Chapple and May[53] on the way in which genetic information may affect social relationships within families showed that the geneticist spent most of the consultation time looking for a diagnosis, explaining the details of genetic inheritance and considering the risks to future offspring. The finding, that psychosocial issues such as stigmatisation, guilt or possible damage to social relationships were rarely discussed,[53] has been upheld in more recent research, suggesting that there is poor communication about genetic risk between relatives in families.[59,60]

Chapple *et al.*[54] propose a number of strategies that can be used when providing genetic counselling. These include: using simple, understandable language giving clear explanations for unfamiliar terms (particularly diagnostic terms) that cannot be avoided. They suggest that careful choice of words, and detailed explanation, not only reduces the risks of 'labelling' and stigmatisation, but may also reduce feelings of fear and confusion and prevent unnecessary anxiety experienced by the individual when they hear unfamiliar medical terms. They also recommend that people are offered simple written information about the disease and given the opportunity to return for further advice if necessary.

ADVANCE CARE PLANNING (ACP)

Research in disclosure of dementia and advance care planning (ACP) has shown that physicians may disclose a diagnosis of dementia openly but not discuss future care needs or end-of-life wishes.[61] If diagnosis is made early, people will have capacity to engage in discussions on prognosis and to be involved in decision-making processes. However, for people experiencing CJD, diagnosis is often made when the disease has progressed significantly.

KEY POINT 12.7

It is essential to engage families and significant others in decision making, particularly related to symptom management, artificial feeding, hydration, and end-of-life care issues (*see* Chapter 6).

Proxy decision making about end-of-life decision is particularly difficult for families and caregivers.[62]

Recommendations have been made by the National Institute for Health and Clinical Excellence[63] that assessment and discussion about a person's physical, psychological, social, spiritual and financial support needs should be undertaken at key points. These key points have been identified as at:

➤ diagnosis
➤ the start, during and end of a specific treatment
➤ relapse
➤ when death is imminent.

The opportunity to discuss ACP with families and caregivers is one way to support them in their grief and distress. ACP could both improve end-of-life care for dying people experiencing CJD and improve the experience of family members involved in end-of-life decision making.

CONCLUSION

Caring for a person experiencing CJD and their family at the end-of-life is complex. It requires sound knowledge about the specific symptoms of the diseases, awareness of the type of stresses that may be experienced by family members and also a general awareness and knowledge of issues and challenges in caring for any person experiencing a dementia syndrome at the end-of-life.

REFERENCES

1 Roberts DJ. The pathophysiology of variant Creutzfeldt-Jakob disease: the hypothesis behind the concerns for blood components and products. *British Journal of Haematology*. 2003; **122**: 3–9.
2 Belay ED, Schonberger LB. The public health impact of prion diseases. *Annual Reviews in Public Health*. 2005; **26**: 191–212.
3 Sikorska B, Liberski PP. Human prion diseases: from kuru to variant Creutzfeldt-Jakob disease. *Subcellular Biochemistry*. 2012; **65**: 457–96.

4 Brown K, Mastrianni JA. The prion diseases. *Journal of Geriatric Psychiatry and Neurology.* 2010; **23**: 277–98.

5 Will RG. Acquired prion disease: iatrogenic CJD, variant CJD, kuru. *British Medical Bulletin.* 2003; **66**: 255–65.

6 National CJD Surveillance Unit. *Creutzfeldt-Jakob Disease Surveillance in the UK.* The National CJD Surveillance Unit, Edinburgh and Department of Infectious and Tropical Diseases, London. 2012. Available at www.cjd.ed.ac.uk (accessed 12 March 2014).

7 Llewellyn CA, Hewitt PE, Knight RSG, *et al.* Possible transfusion of variant Creutzfeldt-Jakob disease by blood transfusion. *Lancet.* 2004; **363**: 422–8.

8 Hewitt PE, Llewellyn CA, Mackenzie J, *et al.* Creutzfeldt-Jakob disease and blood transfusion: results of the UK Transfusion Medicine Epidemiology Review study. *Vox Sanguinis.* 2006; **91**: 221–30.

9 Ironside JW. Variant Creutzfeldt-Jakob disease. *Haemophilia.* 2010; **16**(Suppl. 5): 175–80.

10 Barnett F, McLean G. Care management of Creutzfeldt-Jakob Disease within the United Kingdom. *Journal of Nursing Management.* 2005; **13**: 111–8.

11 Ludlam C, Turner M. Managing the risk of transmission of variant Creutzfeldt-Jakob Disease by blood products. *British Journal of Haematology.* 2005; **132**: 13–24.

12 Will RG, Ironside JW, Zeidler M, *et al.* A new variant of Creutzfeldt-Jakob disease in the UK. *Lancet.* 1996; **347**: 921–5.

13 Will RG, Zeidler M, Stewart GE, *et al.* Diagnosis of new variant Creutzfeldt-Jakob disease. *Annals of Neurology.* 2000; **47**: 575–82.

14 Heath CA, Cooper SA, Murray K, *et al.* Validation of diagnostic criteria for variant Creutzfeldt-Jakob disease. *Annals of Neurology.* 2010; **67**: 761–70.

15 MacKay GH, Knight RSG, Ironside JW. The molecular epidemiology of variant CJD. *Molecular Epidemiology and Genetics.* 2011; **2**: 217–27.

16 Verdrager J. Kuru and 'new variant' CJD. *South East Asian Journal of Tropical Medicine and Public Health.* 1997; **28**: 535–40.

17 Ironside JW, Head MW. Variant Creutzfeldt-Jakob disease and its transmission by blood. *Journal of Thrombosis and Haemostasis.* 2003; **1**: 1479–86.

18 Knight R. Clinical features and diagnosis of human prion diseases. *Future Neurology.* 2008; **3**: 473–81.

19 Knight R. Creutzfeldt-Jakob disease: a rare cause of dementia in elderly persons. *Clinical Infectious Diseases.* 2006; **43**: 340–6.

20 Andrews NJ. *Incidence of variant Creutzfeldt-Jakob disease diagnoses and deaths in the UK January 1994–December 2011.* London: Statistics Unit, Centre for Infections, Health Protection Agency; 2012.

21 de Pedro Cuesta J, Ruiz Tovar M, Ward H, *et al.* Sensitivity to biases of case-control studies on medical procedures, particularly surgery and blood transfusion, and risk of Creutzfeldt-Jakob disease. *Neuroepidemiology.* 2012; **39**: 1–18.

22 Edgeworth JA, Farmer M, Sicilia A, *et al.* Detection of prion infection in variant Creutzfeldt-Jakob disease: a blood-based assay. *Lancet.* 2011; **377**: 487–93.

23 Stride P, Hunter J, Bailey M. Nursing patients with Creutzfeldt-Jakob disease. Are you at risk? *Australian Nursing Journal.* 2009; **17**: 30–2.

24 van Everbroeck B, Quoilin S, Boons J, *et al.* A prospective study of CSF markers in 250 patients with possible Creutzfeldt-Jakob disease. *Journal of Neurology and Neurosurgical Psychiatry.* 2003; **74**: 1210–4.

25 Zeidler M, Johnstone EC, Bamber RW, *et al.* New variant Creutzfeldt-Jakob disease: psychiatric features. *Lancet.* 1997; **350**: 908–10.

26 Brown P, Brandel J, Sato T, *et al.* Iatrogenic Creutzfeldt-Jakob disease, final assessment. *Emerging Infectious Diseases.* 2012; **8**: 901–7.

27 Lorains JW, Henry C, Agbamu DA. Variant CJD in an elderly patient. *Lancet.* 2001; **457**: 1339.

28 Henry C, Lowman A, Will RG. Creutzfeldt-Jakob disease in elderly people. *Age and Ageing.* 2002; **31**: 7–10.

29 Douglas MJ, Campbell H, Will RG. *Patients with New Variant Creutzfeldt-Jakob Disease and Their Families: care and information needs.* Edinburgh: National Surveillance Unit for CJD; 1999.

30 Spencer MD, Knight RSG, Will RG. First hundred cases of variant Creutzfeldt-Jakob disease: retrospective case note review of early psychiatric and neurological features. *British Medical Journal.* 2002; **324**: 1479–82.

31 de Vries K. Nursing patients with variant Creutzfeldt-Jakob disease. *European Journal of Palliative Care.* 2003; **10**: 9–12.

32 de Vries K, Sque MR, Bryan K, *et al.* Variant Creutzfeldt-Jakob disease: need for mental health and palliative care team collaboration. *International Journal of Palliative Nursing.* 2003; **9**: 512–20.

33 Bailey B, Aranda S, Quinn K, *et al.* Creutzfeldt-Jakob disease: extending palliative care nursing knowledge. *International Journal of Palliative Nursing.* 2000; **6**: 131–9.

34 Barnett F. Nursing patients with variant Creutzfeldt-Jakob disease at home. *British Journal of Community Nursing.* 2002; **7**: 445–50.

35 Prout K. Help at hand for people dealing with prion disease. *Nursing Times.* 2000; **96**: 39–40.

36 World Health Organization. *Cancer Pain Relief.* 2nd ed. Geneva: World Health Organization; 1996.

37 Vargas-Schaffer G. Is the WHO analgesic ladder still valid? *Canadian Family Physician.* 2010; **56**: 514–7.

38 Douglas S, James I, Ballard C. Non-pharmacological interventions in dementia. *Advances in Psychiatric Treatment.* 2004; **10**: 171–9.

39 Leung L. From ladder to platform: a new concept for pain management. *Journal of Primary Health Care.* 2012; **4**: 254–8.

40 Burgener SC, Berger B. Measuring perceived stigma in persons with progressive neurological disease: Alzheimer's dementia and Parkinson's disease *Dementia.* 2008; **7**: 31–53.

41 Garand L, Lingler JH, Conner KO, *et al.* Diagnostic labels, stigma, and participation in research related to dementia and mild cognitive impairment. *Gerontological Nursing.* 2009; **2**: 112–21.

42 Gullette MM. Overcoming the terror of forgetfulness: why America's escalating fear of memory loss is dangerous to our human relations, our mental health, and public policy. *Healing Ministry.* 2011; **18**: 21–5.

43 French SL, Floyd M, Wilkins S, *et al.* The Fear of Alzheimer's Disease Scale: a new measure designed to assess anticipatory dementia in older adults. *International Journal of Geriatric Psychiatry.* 2012; **27**: 521–8.

44 Robinson C, Bottorff J. When a desired home death does not occur: the consequences of broken promises. *Journal of Palliative Medicine.* 2013; **16**: 875–80.

45 Gessert CE, Forbes S, Bern-Klug M. Planning end-of-life care for patients with dementia: roles of families and health professionals. *Omega.* 2001; **42**: 273–91.

46 Forbes S, Bern-Klug M, Gessert C. End-of life decision making for nursing home residents with dementia. *Journal of Nursing Scholarship.* 2000; **32**: 251–8.

47 Lewis M, Hepburn K, Narayan S, *et al.* Decision making by family caregivers of elders experiencing dementia. *American Journal of Alzheimer's Disease and Other Dementias.* 2000; **15**: 361–6.

48 Hirschman K, Kapo J, Karlawish J. Why doesn't a family member of a person with advanced dementia use a substituted judgment when making a decision for that person? *American Journal of Geriatric Psychiatry.* 2006; **14**: 659–67.

49 Chan D, Livingston G, Jones L, *et al.* Grief reactions in dementia carers: a systematic review. *International Journal of Geriatric Psychiatry.* 2013; **28**: 1–17.

50 Rando TA. Anticipatory mourning: a review and critique of the literature. In: Rando TA, editor. *Clinical Dimensions of Anticipatory Mourning: theory and practice in working with the dying, their loved ones, and their caregivers.* Champaign, IL: Research Press; 2000. pp. 17–50.

51 Marwit SJ, Meuser TM. Development of a short form inventory to assess grief in caregivers of dementia patients. *Death Studies.* 2005; **29**: 191–205.

52 de Vries K, McChrystal J. Using attachment theory to improve the care of people with dementia. *International Journal of Work Organisation and Emotion.* 2010; **3**: 287–301.

53 Chapple A, May C. Genetic knowledge and family relationships: two case studies. *Health & Social Care in the Community.* 1996; **4**: 166–71.

54 Chapple A, Campion P, May C. Clinical terminology: anxiety and confusion amongst families undergoing genetic counselling. *Patient Education and Counselling.* 1997; **32**: 81–91.

55 Wiseman M, Dancyger C, Michie S. Communicating genetic risk information within families: a review. *Familial Cancer.* 2010; **9**: 691–703.

56 Harder A, Gregor AT, Wirth F, *et al.* Early age of onset in fatal familial insomnia: two novel cases and review of the literature. *Journal of Neurology.* 2004; **251**: 715–24.

57 Finkler K, Skrzynia C, Evans JP. The new genetics and its consequences for family, kinship, medicine and medical genetics. *Social Science & Medicine.* 2003; **57**: 403–12.

58 Finkler K. Family, kinship, memory and temporality in the age of the new Genetics. *Social Science & Medicine.* 2005; **61**: 1059–71.

59 Forrest K, Simpson SA, Wilson BJ, *et al.* To tell or not to tell: barriers and facilitators in family communication about genetic risk. *Departments of Clinical Genetics.* 2003; **64**: 317–26.

60 Wilson BJ, Forrest K, van Teijlingen ER, *et al.* Family communication about genetic risk: the little that is known. *Community Genetics.* 2004; **7**: 15–24.

61 Laakkonen ML, Raivio MM, Eloniemi-Sulkava U, *et al.* Disclosure of dementia diagnosis and the need for advance care planning in individuals with Alzheimer's disease. *Journal of the American Geriatric Society.* 2008; **56**: 2156–7.

62 Livingston G, Leavey G, Manela M, *et al.* Making decisions for people with dementia who lack capacity: qualitative study of family carers in UK. *British Medical Journal* (Overseas & Retired Doctors Edition). 2010; **341**: 494–4.

63 National Institute for Clinical Excellence (NICE). *Improving Supportive and Palliative Care for Adults with Cancer.* London: National Institute for Clinical Excellence; 2004.

TO LEARN MORE

- Cooper J. Caring Relationships. In: *Palliative Care within Mental Health: principles and philosophy.* London/New York: Radcliffe Publishing; 2012. pp. 80–96.
- CJD Support Group Network. Available at: www.cjdsupport.org.au
- Oliver D. The special needs of the neurological patient. In: Cooper J, editor. *Stepping into Palliative Care 2: care and practice.* 2nd ed. Oxford: Radcliffe Publishing; 2006. pp. 225–38.
- Penson J. Bereavement. In: Cooper J, editor. *Stepping into Palliative Care 2: care and practice.* 2nd ed. Oxford: Radcliffe Publishing; 2006. pp. 200–7.
- Penson J. Living with loss. In: *Palliative Care within Mental Health: principles and philosophy.* London/New York: Radcliffe Publishing; 2012. pp. 238–50.
- Williams-Evans S, Broome B. End of life. In: *Palliative Care within Mental Health: principles and philosophy.* London/New York: Radcliffe Publishing; 2012. pp. 220–37.

CHAPTER 13

Euthanasia, assisted suicide and mental health

David Jeffrey

INTRODUCTION

In recent years, in the United Kingdom (UK), there have been a number of widely publicised cases of people in particularly difficult circumstances who have requested a hastened death to end their suffering. Over the same period, there have been a number of attempts in the UK to legalise euthanasia or assisted suicide (AS). The debate over legalisation has become polarised and has focused on the role of doctors in end-of-life care and the modern view of life as personal property; implying that people have a right to choose the timing and manner of their death. Proponents of this view argue that people choosing euthanasia or AS are merely exercising their autonomy.

This chapter will focus on euthanasia and AS with particular reference to mental health issues. There are a small number of people for whom a sense of control is so important that they would like their life to end sooner rather than later and so request euthanasia or AS. In the UK, there is at present no legal 'right to die', nor any obligation or duty for others to end the life of the person who requests help to die. Indeed, aiding or encouraging another person to commit suicide is against the law. Respect for an individual's autonomy must be balanced with the needs of many other vulnerable people who may be harmed if AS were to be legalised.[1] Healthcare professionals and politicians are concerned with the potential adverse effects of legalisation on vulnerable groups including the mentally ill and disabled. Consequently, they have opposed changes in the current law that prohibits both euthanasia and assisted suicide in Britain. Lord Falconer in England and Margo Macdonald in Scotland have expressed their intention to present Bills in the future to legalise assisted death, so it is vital that all healthcare professionals should consider their professional role and the emotional impact of active participation in a person's death. It is worrying to note that in Belgium, where euthanasia is legal, nurses who were involved in administering lethal drugs in about half the cases of euthanasia in institutional settings were rarely involved in the decision-making process.[2]

KEY POINT 13.1

Palliative care depends on effective teamwork. To ignore the views of colleagues results in poor end-of-life care.

REFLECTIVE PRACTICE EXERCISE 13.1

Time: 15 minutes
- How do you feel your professional practice would be affected by the legalisation of euthanasia and AS?
- How would you feel about taking part in hastening another person's death?
- What do you think might be the effect on intra- inter-disciplinary teamwork if euthanasia and AS were legalised in Britain?

This chapter examines how healthcare professionals can respond to a request to 'help me to die'. The terms of the debate should be clarified from the outset. A professional who intentionally kills a person by the administration of drugs, at the person's voluntary and competent request, is carrying out euthanasia. If the professional helps a person to commit suicide by providing lethal doses of drugs for self–administration, at that person's voluntary and competent request, then he or she is participating in assisted suicide (AS).[3]

'Hastened death' includes both euthanasia and AS, as defined above, since in both the intention of the healthcare professional is to cause the death of the person and the treatment prescribed is lethal.

Confusion exists in the distinction between withdrawing or withholding futile treatments and causing death. There is a tendency to overlook the fact that diseases such as cancer or advanced heart failure have a lethal capacity that cannot be resisted indefinitely. To withdraw life-prolonging treatments when these are not of benefit to the individual is to recognise the limits of a professional's power, allowing the dying person to die because of their underlying disease. This is clinically, ethically and legally different from deliberate ending life as in euthanasia or AS.[4]

The arguments for and against legalisation are beyond the scope of this chapter but are briefly summarised in Table 13.1, and readers can learn more from the books cited, which present opposing views.

TABLE 13.1 The euthanasia debate[5]

Pro-euthanasia arguments	Anti-euthanasia arguments
• Right to die	• Sanctity of life
• Relief of suffering	• Infers some lives are worth less than others
• Autonomy	• Slippery slope
• Choice	• Not in person's best interests
• Possible to regulate	• Exposes vulnerable people to pressure to end their lives
• Saving resources	• Regulation not practical
• It happens anyway	• Too much power to doctors
• Is death a bad thing?	• Palliative care is a better alternative

---

> **KEY POINT 13.2**
>
> The public, the individual, family and many professionals misunderstand palliative care.

The World Health Organization defines palliative care as follows:

> Palliative care is an approach that improves the quality of life of patients and their families facing the problems associated with life-threatening illness, through the prevention and relief of suffering by means of early identification and impeccable assessment and treatment of pain and other problems, physical, psychosocial and spiritual.[6]

This chapter looks at the practical implications of a request for euthanasia or AS, people's suffering, their families and the professionals caring for them.

MENTAL ILL-HEALTH AND REQUESTS FOR A HASTENED DEATH

Psychiatrists have regarded suicide a result of mental ill-health and irrational. Over 90% of people who commit suicide have diagnosable mental health problems, and most individuals who attempt suicide have mental health problems. A number of mental health problems are associated with suicide (Box 13.1).[7]

BOX 13.1 Mental health problems associated with suicide[7]

- Depression
- Personality disorders
- Alcohol and substance use
- Anxiety disorders
- Schizophrenia
- Bipolar disorders
- Post-traumatic mood disorders.

Kelly cautions that we only have a limited understanding of the underlying causes of common mental health problems, including depression and schizophrenia. In the individual's case, it is very difficult to predict whether therapy will be effective and impossible to say which individuals will have a spontaneous remission.[8]

People who desire death during terminal ill-health are usually suffering from a treatable depression.[9]

> **KEY POINT 13.3**
>
> A request for hastened death is most often a cry for help and a sign of depression. If people do receive appropriate palliative care, their wish for death usually disappears.

A wish to die is not stable over time but fluctuates, often in response to a person's social situation; assessing the request is particularly complex.[10] Some people experiencing terminal ill-health suffer from a combination of post-traumatic stress disorder and depression described as post-traumatic mood disorder, which is associated with suicidal behaviour.[11,12]

Healthcare professionals have a general obligation to prevent suicide. They are permitted to intervene to prevent loss of life due to mental health problems.[13] Good practice demands careful assessment of anyone known to have suicidal thoughts, plans or behaviours.

SELF-ASSESSMENT EXERCISE 13.1

Time: 5 minutes

Consider the reason why some people request euthanasia or assisted suicide.

LOSS OF SELF, AUTONOMY AND DIGNITY

There is a lack of reliable evidence as to how most dying people feel about euthanasia and AS. Such evidence that does exist indicates that requests relate to feelings of 'disintegration', resulting from a loss of function, a feeling of loss of control and a loss of close personal relationships.[14] As Chochinov observes:

> How patients perceive themselves to be valued is an important part of their dignity. People who feel that life is no longer worth living are more likely to believe that they are just a burden to others.[15]

If healthcare professionals can affirm that the person does matter, the person's sense of dignity will be preserved.[15]

There is a wide variety of opinions as to what constitutes individual autonomy. A narrow view of autonomy equates it with free choice, implying a right to die. A broader view is that autonomy involves a reflective component that takes account of a person's choice on the lives of others, thus considering the effect of legalisation of euthanasia on more vulnerable people.[4]

AMBIVALENCE AND FEAR OF THE FUTURE

The request for euthanasia or AS can alter with changes in an individual's social circumstances independent of the severity of their disease. Moreover, research indicates that fear of future possibilities such as pain, lack of quality of life or lack of hope may influence the request. What is most significant in these findings is that the wishes for euthanasia/AS were ambivalent and liable to change with time.[16] This ambivalence between wishing a hastened death and clinging to life is common as death approaches. Other examples of psychological ambivalence at this time include between hope and despair, certainty and uncertainty, the will to live and the wish to die. Given this uncertainty, the euthanasia wish might represent a need to control pain, feelings of hopelessness or a way to cope with the fear of pain. Viewed as a coping strategy, such wishes might generate an experience of an inner freedom of choice, of having the option of requesting euthanasia/AS. These findings concur with the feelings of many in Oregon who supported AS legislation as a 'safety net'.[17]

EXPERIENCE OF COUNTRIES WHERE EUTHANASIA/AS ARE LEGAL

It is appropriate at this stage to examine the experience of countries where euthanasia and/or AS are legal. Euthanasia is now legal in the Netherlands, Belgium and Luxembourg. Assisted suicide is legal in the Netherlands, Switzerland and the states of Oregon and Washington in the United States of America.

The Netherlands

In the Netherlands, where both euthanasia and AS are legal, the most frequent reasons for requesting euthanasia or AS were pointless suffering, loss of dignity and weakness. In a study, 13% of people withdrew the request and in 12% of cases, the physicians refused the person's request.[18]

Suffering

Suffering is a subjective concept, familiar to everyone but difficult to define. It encompasses factors that diminish quality of life, a perception of distress and is a feeling of a life not worth living.[19] Suffering poses a threat to the integrity of the person and comprises much more than symptom distress. Psychosocial, existential and spiritual aspects of a person's experience at the end-of-life can all contribute to their suffering. Suffering experienced by the individual extends to both the family and healthcare professionals. The family may empathise with the individual and suffer with her or his pain; they may have fears of hastening death by giving medication. There can be conflicts of responsibility between care of the individual and that of dependent children. Prolonged dying is stressful for families and can lead to emotional fatigue.

If doctors perceive suffering as a problem to 'manage', the process of dying could be reduced to a progression of problems to confront. Preoccupation with the clinical aspects of the disease may distance the professional carers from engaging closely. Not every professional feels comfortable in engaging with the psychological complexities of communicating with dying people. In some cases, the person's request for euthanasia/AS may be an indication that other professionals have despaired of them.

KEY POINT 13.4

It would be unwise to give doctors the power to issue lethal prescriptions for assisted suicide if they lack the empathy to explore the suffering of a dying person.[4]

Doctors are centrally involved in euthanasia and AS and the emotional and psychological effects on the participating doctor can be substantial.[20]

The practice of euthanasia in the Netherlands is an example of the impossibility of resisting a widening interpretation and application of the law, the so-called slippery slope. The Netherlands has moved from euthanasia and AS for unrelieved suffering to euthanasia for being 'tired of life', to euthanasia for dementia, to euthanasia for neonates and euthanasia without consent.[21]

Oregon

In a study of 988 terminally ill people in the USA, 60% supported euthanasia/AS in a hypothetical situation but only 10% considered euthanasia/AS for themselves. Factors associated with those being *less* likely to consider euthanasia/AS were feeling valued, being over 65 or being African-American. Factors associated with being *more* likely to consider euthanasia/AS were depressive symptoms or perceived feelings of being a burden to carers, and pain. At follow-up interview, half of the terminally ill people who had considered AS for themselves had changed their minds.[22]

In Oregon, studies of dying people have shown that about half would like the option of AS to be available for possible future use. However, only 10% of these people seriously consider AS, only 1% specifically request it, and only 0.1% actually take a lethal prescription.[23]

People in Oregon who asked for AS tended to have strong personalities, were better educated, lived in urban settings, had been in a position of responsibility in life, and found being cared for intolerable. Their most important concerns were loss of autonomy, inability to participate in pleasurable activity and loss of dignity. Inadequate pain control and self-perceived burden were less common concerns.[17,24]

Some people have dropped the word 'suicide' in the context of hastened death because of the connection with irrationality and its emotional charge. The Oregon Department of Human Services, which oversees the Oregon Death with Dignity Act, no longer refers to a death under this law as assisted suicide or physician-assisted suicide.[25]

FEELING A BURDEN
SELF-ASSESSMENT EXERCISE 13.2

> **Time: 5 minutes**
> Think of what could be perceived as types of burdens on a family whose loved one is dying.

A sense of being a burden on others can result in feelings of guilt, distress and a diminished sense of self and is a common motive for requesting euthanasia.[26] The types of burden can include:
➤ the strains of caregiving
➤ responsibility for making difficult treatment decisions
➤ financial difficulty.

In a qualitative study of terminally ill men, 'burden to others' emerged as a concern for the men in different phases of their ill-health.[27] One phase was 'living while dying', which was characterised by a need to minimise burden on others. Later, 'anticipating a transition to active dying', which was marked by a concern as to the impact of their death and the dying process on others. The third phase expressed by people in this study was 'completing preparations', which was viewed as a way of reducing the burden on their families after their death.[27]

Singer found that a person's feelings of being a burden to their family arose in the context of three situations:
1   providing physical care
2   witnessing the death
3   decision making for life-sustaining treatment.[28]

Other important reasons for requesting euthanasia or AS include:
➤ depression
➤ hopelessness
➤ need for social support.

➤ dementia or the fear of dementia
➤ psychological distress

These issues will now be looked at in more detail.

DEPRESSION

Suicidal intent is regarded as a sign of mental disturbance. Whether suicide can be rational is a philosophical question beyond the scope of this chapter. However, mental health professionals face a dramatic change in role should suicide be reinterpreted as a rational choice. While a right to die already exists since the decriminalisation of suicide, a right to be killed by someone else involves not only a change of law but a huge moral leap.[29]

In people suffering with painful, disabling and terminal ill-health, depression is common and may underlie suicidal thoughts, which can generally be relieved by appropriate support and by effective treatments. Many professionals do not recognise depression, or know how to assess for its presence in people experiencing terminally ill-health.[9,10,22,30,31]

KEY POINT 13.5

Depression is a subtle condition that may be difficult to diagnose. If the diagnosis is missed, then all 'safeguards' in any legislation of euthanasia are ineffective.

Even when recognised, some professionals take the view that in people experiencing terminal ill-health, 'understandable depression' cannot be treated or is not 'real' depression. Therefore, in this group of people depression often goes untreated and in some cases in the Netherlands, AS or euthanasia is provided even when depression is present.[32]

Ganzini and her colleagues examined the prevalence of depression and anxiety in people requesting AS in Oregon. They had a cohort of 58 Oregonians who had requested AS. Fifteen had clinical depression and 13 anxiety. Forty-two people died by the end of their study, 18 received a supply of lethal drugs, 15 did not meet the criteria for a diagnosis of depression. Worryingly, three people who did have clinical depression died by ingesting the lethal drug.[33]

Perhaps the commonest dilemma facing professionals in requests for euthanasia or AS are people whose judgement is affected by mild depression, mild cognitive impairment and pressure from others. Additionally, the wish for euthanasia or AS changes over time in a large proportion of terminally ill people and this ambivalence is associated with depression.

DEMENTIA

Mental health services are involved with the assessment, diagnosis and treatment of people experiencing dementia (*see* Chapters 11,12). As the disease progresses, institutional care usually becomes necessary, resulting in a huge demand for resources, which will challenge the sustainability of health and social care services.[29]

People fear dementia in part because they foresee inevitable misery and degradation and do not see a capacity for resilience and adaptation.[34]

KEY POINT 13.6

Researchers found that people experiencing dementia rate their own quality of life as higher than the views of their families and carers.[35]

Those campaigning to legalise assisted dying have focused on a perceived loss of dignity at the end-of-life, particularly in relation to dementia. They imply that dementia in the terminal stage is necessarily undignified. This view could extend to devalue the status of all people with dementia and risks perpetuating the poor standards of care which have been reported in some institutions. Being dependent on others does not necessarily imply a loss of dignity, since we are all dependent on others and this dependence is part of our humanity. There is no straightforward correlation between quality of life and measureable clinical variables in dementia. Depression also occurs in people experiencing dementia and detection is difficult.

Kitwood reminds us to keep the person as the central focus and if he or she is experiencing dementia, they still have experiences and thoughts just like everyone else. The worst indignity that professionals can instigate is to deny people experiencing dementia their personhood.[36]

KEY POINT 13.7

Palliative care for people experiencing dementia is a recent concept and aims to improve quality of life without hastening death.

Such care can prevent the undignified death portrayed by euthanasia campaigners.[37]

People experiencing dementia might feel a pressure for self-sacrifice. Baroness Mary Warnock was reported as saying that people experiencing dementia were a burden on their families and a waste of NHS resources.[38] This ignores the huge gains derived by families and professionals in caring for ill relatives. Caring is a reciprocal activity which benefits both the giver and the receiver of care.

With these insights into the complexities of the interacting motives for requesting euthanasia or AS, we now need to consider how to respond to the person making the request for a hastened death.

RESPONDING TO A REQUEST FOR EUTHANASIA/AS

In countries that have legalised euthanasia and/or assisted suicide, mental health assessment of people wishing a hastened death is recommended but rarely occurs. In the Netherlands, psychiatrists are only involved in 4% of all physician-assisted deaths.[32] In Oregon, where AS is legal, with the passage of time it has become increasingly uncommon for people requesting AS to have any psychiatric assessment. In 2012, of the 77 people who took the lethal prescription in Oregon only two were referred for formal psychological or mental health evaluation. Moreover, it is rare for there to be a doctor present when the person commits suicide; the prescribing doctor was present at the time of ingestion in less than 10% of deaths.[25]

> ### Case Study 13.1
> Morag (32) is a primary school teacher and is married to Tom, a computer programmer. She has two children, Martha (4) and Gabriel (2). She is experiencing advanced breast cancer with bone and liver spread. Morag has declined further palliative chemotherapy. She asks her general practitioner, 'Please can you help me to die?'

REFLECTIVE PRACTICE EXERCISE 13.1

> **Time: 10 minutes**
> * Think of the possible reasons for Morag's request.
> * How would you respond to Morag's plea?

It is critical that the professionals possess the necessary skills to identify ambivalence. Given the many possible meanings of a wish for euthanasia/AS, it is crucial that the professional assesses the request in a sophisticated manner and does not respond to the person's wishes at face value.

ASSESSMENT

Assessment in end-of-life care depends upon continuity of care by a multi-professional team and is an ongoing dynamic activity. It is unrealistic to imagine that a single consultation with a person could reveal all the factors behind a request for euthanasia or AS. It may take days or even weeks to establish a sufficiently trusting relationship with a person to allow discussion of these intimate concerns. Compounding these difficulties is the lack of time, continuity and the fact that many individuals have a number of attending professionals involved in their care.

The assessment of the euthanasia/AS request may even create a barrier that subtly alters the professional–individual relationship; paradoxically, this might impair the possibility of discussing the hopes and fears driving the request.

The meaning behind the request is not confined to the reality of physical disintegration or suffering from the effects of her or his disease, but includes fears and existential concerns with desires for connectedness, care and respect. So professionals should respond to the euthanasia request by not merely attending to issues of the individual's competency in their decision making but also sensitively exploring the underlying reasons for the wish for euthanasia/AS.[39]

First steps in exploring feelings

The first step is to establish connection with the person. This is a time when the professional sits down and is prepared to listen with empathy. It is totally unhelpful to dismiss the request by saying, 'Oh, you know I can't do that. It is against the law.' There will be an appropriate moment later when it will be possible to say, 'You know that euthanasia is against the law and I can't help you with that … but let us look at what we can do to help …'

Instead, the professional should acknowledge the difficulty of the situation: 'That is a difficult question, we need to spend time to find out a bit more, can you please tell me what you mean by help to die?'

Clarification of ambiguities such as 'help to die', exploration of the reasons for the request and a genuine attempt to understand some of the distress the person is going through are integral to the assessment. There can be few fixed rules of how to respond to a person in such distress other than to follow their agenda. This communication requires the professional to be sensitive to cues that the person offers.

SELF-ASSESSMENT EXERCISE 13.3

Time: 5 minutes
What cues would you be looking for?

Cues may signal unrelieved pain, depression or fears of loss of control. The professional needs to make the person aware of the intra- inter-disciplinary team and perhaps suggest another team member who might also be able to help in discussions.

Once it has been clarified that the person is requesting euthanasia or AS, the professional needs to explore:
➤ the person's reasons for the request
➤ feelings about the situation

➤ the person's competence to make a decision
➤ to screen for underlying mental health problems.[40]

In addition, palliative care is concerned with supporting the family so professionals need to be aware of the family's position, and to be sure that they are not exerting any pressure on the person to choose euthanasia.

Mental capacity and competence

A test for mental capacity is a negative one in that competence has to be disproved for a finding of incapacity.[41] There are three important requirements in the common law test of capacity. The person must be able to:
1 comprehend and retain information
2 weigh the information and reach a decision
3 communicate their decision.[41]

The test is context-specific, which means that it focuses on the person's ability to make a decision about the question at hand.

The individual must have mental capacity before a request for euthanasia/AS can be considered. Some professionals know little about capacity assessments and fail to recognise that a person lacks capacity. The assessment of decision-making capacity for people experiencing terminal ill-health has not been researched. Furthermore, bias in the mental capacity assessment may occur because those who support euthanasia/AS as an option may be more willing to find the person's judgement unimpaired.[42]

Macleod asserts that assessment of competency in a sustained wish to die; depressive symptoms, dementia and unbearable suffering in the terminally ill are clinically difficult tasks:

> As yet psychiatry does not have the expertise to 'select' those whose wish
> for hastened death is rational, humane, and healthy.[43]

Rarely in those societies where euthanasia and/or AS are legal are mental health professionals involved in the decision making. Non-specialists usually fulfil this role. This raises significant concerns regarding the accuracy of mental health assessment in the terminally ill, where capacity may be intermittent or fluctuating. Capacity can also be eroded by delirium or depression, both conditions which can be difficult to diagnose in the terminally ill.[43,44]

A survey showed that 64% of British psychiatrists felt a psychiatric assessment of a request for hastened death to be important, but only 35% would be willing to carry out such an assessment.[45] Ganzini found that among Oregon psychiatrists only 6% felt confident that a single assessment could enable them to decide whether or not mental health problems were influencing a person's request.[46]

Professionals who are opposed to euthanasia/AS may not wish to take any part in the process. The persistent emotional distress of the person making the request can also affect a professional who is not equipped to respond effectively. A professional with limited mental health training may be overwhelmed by the person's emotional distress and may be inclined to favour euthanasia or AS. Research suggests that an attitude that conveys the professional's approval of the wish for euthanasia/AS may even encourage the person to request a hastened death.[47]

Some mental health professionals consider that assisting suicide is incompatible with their role of trying to prevent it by effective treatment. As professionals who specialise in the management of suicide, they are well aware that the request to die is a communication that has different interpretations.

KEY POINT 13.8

It may be that in requesting to die, a person is looking to be given a reason to live. Even if they were not, professionals would still want to offer care, support and effective relief of distress.

ADVANCE DIRECTIVES (LIVING WILLS)

Advance directives are a way of allowing people to state their preferences for their future care and influencing how medical decisions are to be made should the person become incompetent in the future. There is legal recognition in many countries for non-treatment directives or living wills. In England and Wales, the Mental Capacity Act 2005 makes provision for advance decisions for refusing life-sustaining treatments prior to losing the ability to communicate, and this is legally binding on doctors. However, advance directives do not apply to euthanasia or AS.[29]

Mental capacity is lost in advanced dementia but if the scope of advance directives is extended to medically assisted death, then how can we be certain that a person no longer deemed to be competent continues to want their life to end? How could they overturn the legal document if they could not express a change of mind? In any case, a change of mind might depend on sensitive professionals picking up a shrug or other non-verbal clue to the person's underlying uncertainty.

As Leeman points out, competent adults have a legal right to refuse life-sustaining treatment even when death will result from their refusal. Mental health professionals are seldom consulted before the person's request for withholding or withdrawal is acted on. Yet it is possible for treatment refusal to be considered irrational at times.[13]

In the Netherlands, advance directives for euthanasia are legally recognised. Despite their legal possibilities, advance directives for euthanasia are rarely complied with and never in people experiencing dementia. It is interesting that they may be taken into account in limiting life-sustaining treatments, which is not what they were intended for.[48,49]

ADMINISTRATION OF EUTHANASIA/AS

In the Netherlands, euthanasia is administered by the doctor injecting a large dose of barbiturate, often followed by a muscle relaxant to paralyse the person, who dies of respiratory failure. In AS, the individual is given an anti-emetic and then drinks an overdose of barbiturate.

It seems certain that if euthanasia and AS were to become legalised in the UK, mental health professionals would be involved in assessment and decision making. There are training implications since professionals in Britain have no specialised knowledge on how to kill patients.

The effects on other individuals and professionals should be considered if euthanasia/AS took place in the same ward or even building as the one in which they receive treatment. The legalisation of euthanasia or AS would threaten the relationships between people and their professional; the risk of losing trust and damaging care is high. The professional–individual relationship is built upon trust.

KEY POINT 13.9

Every clinician needs to reflect on their practice and consider whether they would be prepared to write the lethal prescription for AS or carry out euthanasia.

They have to imagine how they would feel if problems occurred during the process, and whether ultimately they would give the lethal injection. It is one matter to indulge in a philosophical debate, but to be involved in giving a lethal injection at the bedside of the dying person is quite a different matter.[4]

ASSISTED SUICIDE TOURISM

About 100 British people have travelled to Switzerland to die by assisted suicide. Debbie Purdy, a woman with multiple sclerosis, was contemplating suicide but wanted to know whether her husband would be prosecuted for helping her to travel to Switzerland.[50] The Director of Public Prosecutions responded with a policy which lists the factors which make a prosecution more likely. Included in the list is if the person did not have the capacity to reach an informed decision to commit suicide.[51] To further understand these factors, *see* the DPP's policy in To Learn More at the end of this chapter.

HUMAN RIGHTS

Diane Pretty, who is experiencing motor neurone disease, argued that, deprived of the right to get help to end her life, she was being subjected to inhuman suffering. She appealed to the Law Lords under the Human Rights Act of 1998. Article 2 states:

> Everyone's right to life shall be protected by law. No one shall be deprived of his life intentionally save in the execution of a sentence of a court following his conviction of a crime for which this penalty is provided by law.[52]

Article 3 also asserts:

No one shall be subjected to torture or to inhuman or degrading treatment or punishment.[52]

The Law Lords concluded that the law did not allow her to get help to take her own life.[53]

RESOURCE IMPLICATIONS

There are ethical dangers in linking the euthanasia and assisted suicide debate to limited healthcare resources. There is a potential here for abuse since palliative care is expensive and euthanasia and AS are not. Legalising euthanasia and AS might change the way in which our society views people experiencing mental health problems. They may become seen as an inconvenience and the lethal prescription as a solution to the challenges and particularly the costs of caring for the vulnerable.[4] Mann warns that there is a risk if AS is legalised:

> there will be social expectations for individuals to choose AS as soon as their physical capabilities decline to a point where they become dependent upon others in an expensive inconvenient way.[54]

MEDICAL POWER

Although this chapter has focused on the role of all healthcare professionals, doctors administer the lethal medication in euthanasia and prescribe the lethal drug in assisted suicide. Their motivation in both situations is to hasten death. Involvement in euthanasia or AS would be, in the view of most doctors, incompatible with the duties and obligations of medical practice, and would disregard their professional codes of duty.[54] At present the authority of doctors is being questioned in many areas of their practice, and it would be illogical to give them the power to assist in killing merely because a person wishes to waive his or her right to life. One of the greatest concerns surrounds the issue of trust. The doctor–person relationship depends upon such trust, and to legalise euthanasia or AS would be to put this in jeopardy. It is not the role of doctors to decide when lives are not worth living nor when suffering is too great to be borne, nor do they have the moral authority to make these sorts of judgement. The great majority of doctors, including psychiatrists, do not want to be involved in euthanasia or AS.

CONCLUSION

Meeting the demands of a vocal minority to legalise euthanasia/AS could expose a vulnerable majority to great harm as a right to die becomes a duty to die. The legalisation of euthanasia could lead to a bureaucratic industry of checks and procedures, diverting resources from person-centred care.[29] At the heart of the debate is a moral issue not about what we can do but about what we ought to do. There is a risk of a slippery slope, where there is a widening application of the law, which cannot easily be prevented since judgements rely on interpretation. Criteria such as dignity, suffering and quality of life are highly subjective and could be stretched to include any degree of discomfort or unhappiness.[29]

As Macrae warns, if screening for mental ill-health in people choosing to die became obligatory, all members of the intra- inter-disciplinary mental health team could become gatekeepers to death.[29]

Sher points out that we do not solve problems by getting rid of the people who have the problem. The humane, but admittedly more difficult, solution to human suffering is to address the problem.[7]

KEY POINT 13.10

A core principle of palliative care is that all people are intrinsically valuable and that their quality of life should be maximised.

Professionals work to heal ill-health and to promote health. When cure is no longer possible, healthcare professionals strive to relieve pain and suffering. When death is imminent and unavoidable, professionals should not 'strive officiously' to keep someone alive, nor should they give burdensome treatments. People in despair need to be supported and reassured about their value. They do not want to have their worst fears confirmed and arrangements made for their death.[4] The suffering of those facing imminent death is worsened by feelings of being a burden on others or by being abandoned by their professional carers. We need to remember that presence, kindness and compassion from an interested professional team have an enormous therapeutic effect on suffering at the end-of-life.

SELF-ASSESSMENT EXERCISE 13.4 (*SEE* ANSWERS ON P. 219)

Time: 5 minutes

Which of the following statements are true and which are false?
   1 Assisted suicide is legal in the UK.
   2 In the Netherlands, euthanasia may be carried out legally on newborn babies with spina bifida.
   3 Assisted suicide is illegal in Belgium.
   4 The majority of doctors in the UK want to legalise euthanasia and AS.
   5 Depression is common in the terminally ill.
   6 Depression is usually easy to diagnose in dying people.
   7 People experiencing dementia must face an undignified death.
   8 Most professionals are comfortable with assessing mental capacity.
   9 Psychiatrists are rarely involved in euthanasia requests in the Netherlands.
  10 Palliative care only applies to people dying of cancer.

REFERENCES

1 George RJD, Finlay IG, Jeffrey D. Legalised euthanasia will violate the rights of vulnerable patients. *British Medical Journal.* 2005; **331**: 684–5.

2 Bilsen JJR, Stichele RHV, Mortier F *et al.* Involvement of nurses in physician-assisted dying. *Journal of Advanced Nursing.* 2004; **47**: 583–91.

3 Matersteedt LJ. Palliative care on the 'slippery slope' towards euthanasia. *Palliative Medicine.* 2003; **17**: 387–92.

4 Jeffrey D. *Against Physician Assisted Suicide: a palliative care perspective.* Oxford: Radcliffe Publishing; 2008.

5 BBC Ethics. Euthanasia and anti-euthanasia arguments. Available at: www.bbc.co.uk/ethics/euthanasia (accessed 12 March 2014).

6 World Health Organization. (2002). *National Cancer Control Programmes: policies and managerial guidelines.* 2nd ed. Geneva. www.who.int/cancer/media/en/408.pdf (accessed 12 March 2014).

7 Sher L. What should we tell medical students and residents about euthanasia and assisted suicide? *Australian and New Zealand Journal of Psychiatry.* 2012; **46**: 87–91.

8 Kelly B, Burnett P, Pelusi D, *et al.* Factors associated with the wish to hasten death: a study of patients with terminal illness. *Psychological Medicine.* 2003; **33**: 75–81.

9 Breibart W, Rosenfield B, Pessin H, *et al.* Depression, hopelessness and desire for hastened death in terminally ill patients with cancer. *Journal of the American Medical Association.* 2000; **284**: 2907–11.

10 Chochinov HM, Wilson KG, Enns M, *et al.* Desire for death in the terminally ill *American Journal of Psychiatry.* 1995; **152**: 1185–91.

11 Sher L. Concept of post-traumatic mood disorder. *Medical Hypotheses.* 2005; **65**: 205–10.

12 Bienvenu OJ, Neufeld KT. Post traumatic stress disorder in medical setting: focus on critically ill. *Current Psychiatric Reports.* 2011; **13**: 3.

13 Leeman CP. Distinguishing among irrational suicide and other forms of hastened death: implications for clinical practice. *Psychosomatics.* 2009; **50**: 185–91.

14 Lavery JV, Boyle B, Dickens BM, *et al.* Origins of the desire for euthanasia and assisted suicide in people with HIV-1 or AIDS: a qualitative study. *Lancet.* 2001; **358**: 362–7.

15 Chochinov HM. Dignity and the essence of medicine; the A, B, C, and D of dignity conserving care. *British Medical Journal.* 2007; **335**: 184–7.

16 Johansen S, Holen J, Kaasa S. Attitudes towards, and wishes for, euthanasia in cancer patients at a palliative medicine unit. *Palliative Medicine.* 2005; **19**: 454–60.

17 Hendin H, Foley K. Physician assisted suicide in Oregon; a medical perspective. *Michigan Law Review.* 2008; **106**: 1613–40.

18 Jansen-van Der Weide MC, Onwuteaka BD, Van Der Wal G. Granted, undecided, withdrawn, and refused requests for euthanasia and physician-assisted suicide. *Archives Internal Medicine.* 2005; **165**: 1698–704.

19 Cherny NI, Coyle C, Foley KM. Suffering in the advanced cancer patient: a definition and taxonomy. *Journal of Palliative Care.* 1994; **10**: 57–70.

20 Stevens KR. Emotional and psychological effects of physician-assisted suicide and euthanasia on participating physicians. *Issues in Law & Medicine.* 2006; **21**: 187–200.

21 Hendin H, Rutenfrans C, Zylicz Z. Physician-assisted suicide and euthanasia in the Netherlands. *Journal of the American Medical Association.* 1997; **277**. 1720–2.

22 Emanuel EJ, Fairclough DL, Emanuel LL. Attitudes and desires related to euthanasia and physician-assisted suicide among terminally ill patients and their caregivers. *Journal of the American Medical Association.* 2000; **284**: 2460–8.

23 Bascom PB, Tolle SW. Responding to requests for physician assisted suicide. *Journal of the American Medical Association.* 2002; **288**: 91–8.

24 *House of Lords Report of the Select Committee on Assisted Dying for the Terminally Ill Bill 2004.* London: Stationery Office; 2005.

25 Oregon Death with Dignity Act. Available at: www.healthoregon.org/dwd (accessed 12 March 2014).

26 McPherson CJ, Wilson KG, Murray MA. Feeling like a burden; exploring the perspectives of patients at the end of life. *Social Science Medicine.* 2007; **64**: 417–27.

27 Vig EK, Pearlman RA. Quality of life while dying: a qualitative study of terminally ill older men. *Journal of American Geriatric Society.* 2003; **51**: 1595–601.

28 Singer P, Martin D, Kelner M. Quality end-of-life care: patients' perspectives. *Journal of the American Medical Association.* 1999; **281**; 163–8.

29 McCrae N, Bloomfield J. Mental health nursing and the debate on assisted dying. *Journal of Psychiatric and Mental Health Nursing.* 2013; **20**: 655–61.

30 Bowers L, Boyle DA. Depression in patients with advanced cancer. *Clinical Journal Oncology Nursing.* 2003; **7**: 281–8.

31 Stiefel R, Die Trill M, Berney A, *et al.* Depression in palliative care: a pragmatic report from the Expert Working Group of the European Association for Palliative Care. *Supportive Care Cancer.* 2001; **9**: 477–88.

32 Groeneward JH, van der Heide A, Tholen AJ, *et al.* Psychiatric consultations with regard to euthanasia or physician-assisted suicide. *General Hospital Psychiatry.* 2004; **26**: 323–30.

33 Ganzini L, Goy ER, Dobscha SK. Prevalence of depression and anxiety in patients requesting physicians' aid in dying: cross-sectional survey. *British Medical Journal.* 2008; **307**: a1682.

34 McCrae N, McCrae C. Singer's standards (letter). *Standpoint.* 2011; **34**: 14–5.

35 Gonzalez-Salvador T, Lykersos CG, Baker A, *et al.* Quality of life in dementia patients in long-term care. *International Journal of Geriatric Psychiatry.* 2000; **15**: 181–9.

36 Kitwood T. *Dementia Reconsidered: the person comes first.* Buckingham: Open University Press; 1997.

37 Hughes JC, Jolley D, Jordan A, *et al.* Palliative care in dementia; issues and evidence. *Advances in Psychiatric Treatment.* 2007; **13**: 251–60.

38 Beckford M. Baroness Warnock: Dementia suffers may have a 'duty to die'. *Daily Telegraph.* 18 September 2008.

39 Mak Y, Elwyn G. Voices of the terminally ill: uncovering the meaning of desire for euthanasia. *Palliative Medicine.* 2005; **19**: 343–50.

40 Scott RV. Why assisted suicide must remain illegal in the UK. *Nursing Standard.* 2012; **26**: 40–8.

41 Stewart C, Peisah C, Draper B. A test for mental capacity to request assisted suicide *Journal of Medical Ethics.* 2010; **37**: 34–9.

42 Fenn DS, Ganzini L. Attitude of Oregon psychologists toward PAS and the Oregon Death with Dignity Act. *Professional Psychology: Research and Practice.* 1999; **30**: 235–44.

43 Macleod AD. Assisted dying in liberalised jurisdictions and the role of psychiatry: a clinician's view. *Australian and New Zealand Journal of Psychiatry.* 2012; **46**: 936–45.

44 Ryan CJ. Playing the ferryman: psychiatry's role in end-of-life decision-making. *Australian and New Zealand Journal of Psychiatry.* 2012; **46**: 932–5.

45 Shah N, Warner J, Blizard B, *et al.* National survey of UK psychiatrists attitudes to euthanasia. *Lancet.* 1998; **352**: 1360.

46 Ganzini L, Fenn DS, Lee MA, *et al.* Attitudes of Oregon psychiatrists towards physician assisted suicide. *American Journal of Psychiatry.* 1996; **153**: 1469–75.

47 Kelly BD. Euthanasia, assisted suicide and psychiatry: a Pandora's box. *British Journal of Psychiatry.* 2002; **181**: 278–9.

48 De Boer ME, Droes R-M, Jonker C, *et al.* Advance directives for euthanasia in dementia: how do they affect resident care in Dutch nursing homes? Experiences of physicians and relatives. *Journal of the American Geriatric Society.* 2011; **59**: 989–96.

49 Hertogh CMPM, de Boer ME, Droes R-M, *et al*. Would we rather lose our life than lose our self? Lessons from the Dutch debate on euthanasia for patients with dementia. *American Journal of Bioethics*. 2007; 7: 48–56.

50 *R (Purdy) v Department of Public Prosecutions* (2009) UK HL 45. Director of Public Prosecutions. *Policy for Prosecution in Respect of Cases of Encouraging or Assisting Suicide 2010*. Available at: www.cps.gov.uk/publications/prosecution/assisted_suicide_policy.html (accessed 12 March 2014).

51 Judgements: *The Queen on the application of Mrs Diane Pretty (Appellant) v Director of Public Prosecutions (Respondent) and Secretary of State for the Home Department. (Interested Part)* House of Lords 29 November 2001 (UKHL 61).

52 Baggini J. *Ethics: The Big Questions*. London: Quercus; 2012.

53 Mann PS. Meanings of death. In: Battin PM, Rhodes R, Slivers A, editors. *Physician Assisted Suicide: expanding the debate*. New York: Routledge; 1998. pp. 9–27.

54 Randall F, Downie R. Assisted suicide and voluntary euthanasia; role contradiction for physicians. *Clinical Medicine*. 2010; **10**: 323–5.

TO LEARN MORE

- Director of Public Prosecutions. *Policy for Prosecution in Respect of Cases of Encouraging or Assisting Suicide*. 2010. Available at: www.cps.gov.uk/publications/prosecution/assisted_suicide_policy.html (accessed 12 March 2014).
- Jeffrey D. *Against Physician Assisted Suicide: a palliative care perspective*. Radcliffe Publishing: Oxford; 2008.
- Warnock M, Macdonald E. *Easeful Death: is there a case for assisted dying?* Oxford: Oxford University Press; 2008.

ANSWERS TO SELF-ASSESSMENT EXERCISE 13.4 (*SEE* P. 216)

1	False
2	True
3	True
4	False
5	True
6	False
7	False
8	False
9	True
10	False

CHAPTER 14

Palliative care and substance use: special considerations

Rose Neild, Peter Athanasos

INTRODUCTION

Alcohol, illegal drugs and prescribed drugs used in excess or in risky circumstances can be considered a substance use problem. Why one person becomes dependent and another does not is a fascinating and complex issue but beyond the scope of this chapter. Here we are concerned with the individual whose substance use has impacted on their health in the long term. Individuals with this problem may have periods of remission but may also relapse at times and require further intensive interventions.

Substance use problems, whilst categorised as mental health issues, can and do co-exist with other mental health problems. The mental health problem may have been caused through chronic substance use. In other cases, the substance use problem is caused by the chronic mental health problem. That is, some people experiencing mental health (e.g. depression) or physical health problems (back pain) may use substances inappropriately to manage symptoms – in other words, to help the person feel better. Therefore, here we have mental health and physical problems that may be caused through excessive use of substances but at the same time may be a way of dealing with physical and mental health problems.

For some people experiencing long-term mental health and/or physical problems, the best way forward is the palliative approach. That is, the aim of treatment is not cure but striving for the best *quality of life* in the time that is left. This contrasts with the detoxification and abstinence-only approach that many health professionals promote.[1] Detoxification describes a treatment whereby a drug or drugs are withdrawn, sometimes using medication to improve safety, reduce symptoms and enhance completion rates of the treatment. The goal is to achieve abstinence. Evidence shows that without additional treatment, relapse following detoxification is very common. The individual might need one or a variety of additional therapeutic interventions, for example cognitive behavioural therapy (CBT), other talking therapies or anti-craving medications.

Despite interventions, some people continue to use substances and over the longer term may develop serious mental and physical health problems. In terms of physical health problems, some, but not all, may lead to terminal ill-health. Individuals and their family need considerable care and support when faced with end-of-life ill-health. Palliative care works alongside the individual and family at all times sustaining the status quo of prolonged substance use, or supporting the person and his or her symptoms through to remission, or supporting the person and family through to death ... and beyond (*see* Chapter 5; also *Palliative Care within Mental Health: principles and philosophy*, Chapters 13, 14).

As the person ages, their ability to tolerate substances may decrease. Consequently, substance use will have an increased impact on their physical and mental health, and increased impact on the family. In this situation, there is a specific need for palliation. Palliation is best understood as a healthcare intervention that focuses on relieving, managing and preventing the suffering of the individual and family. Communication and co-ordination with other professionals involved with the individual and consultation of additional specialist professionals as required will prevent unnecessary complications arising.

Substance use is a vast subject and covers all age groups. Consideration of it as a whole is outside the scope of this chapter. Here we concentrate on the terminally ill individual and the care and intervention required for physical health, mental health and substance use.

SUBSTANCE USE – THE OLDER PERSON

Substance use problems are common in the general population and can commonly co-occur with other mental health and physical health problems. Importantly for the individual receiving palliative care, they may not have been identified prior to presentation for treatment.[2] A large number of people from a wide range of backgrounds use substances. In the past, substance use disorders have been identified in far fewer numbers amongst older people compared to the general population. This has led to the misconception that individuals 'age out' of substance use problems. Our understanding has changed. Substance use is now recognised as an important risk for the older person.[2] Furthermore, in Western society, substance use peaked amongst the 'baby boomer' generation who were aged 35–54 years in 2000. As this cohort continues into older age, increased substance use in older people is anticipated.[2]

SUBSTANCE USE PROBLEMS IN CONTEXT

The increased understanding of substance use problems that occurred throughout the twentieth century has led to substantial research and treatment developments. Our understanding has evolved from a moralistic viewpoint at the beginning of the twentieth century (substance disorders occur to those with weak or bad characters who make poor choices) to our present, more complex understanding of the interplay of:

➤ genetic factors
➤ psychological factors
➤ environmental factors.

This evolution of understanding has led to significant changes in intervention.[3] The risk of terminal ill-health in the older person is further increased by the high prevalence of blood-borne viral infections. Such infections may lead to palliative care presentations at a premature age. Moreover, high levels of heavy tobacco and alcohol use amongst older people increase the risks of premature presentations to palliative care services. There are well recognised medical risks of excessive substance use, including:

➤ hepatic
➤ renal
➤ and endocrine disease.

In addition, there is increased risk of a range of cancers and these factors also increase the likelihood that the older person will present to palliative care services.[4,5] These factors may have a substantial effect on the assessment and management as part of the palliative care plan. In addition, these issues may have a substantial effect on how the care plan may be implemented.

BIOLOGICAL CONSIDERATIONS

People with a history of psychoactive drug use may present a range of challenges to palliative care professionals. In the event that the substance use problem is historical rather than current, there may still be residual medical complications of previous use.[6,7] These residual complications may result from chronic infective processes such as hepatitis C and/or human immunodeficiency virus (HIV) and, while they are often a consequence of drug use, may also be unrelated. Complications of chronic substance use problems might include:

➤ cardiac compromise (such as alcohol-related cardiomyopathy)
➤ hepatic compromise (which may be secondary to alcohol use problems, chronic infective hepatitis, other metabolic disorders or a combination of these factors)
➤ pulmonary compromise.[6,7,8,9,10,11]

All body systems may be affected by ongoing substance use and produce co-occurring medical problems (comorbidity). The situation is further complicated by polypharmacy – interactions between multiple medications, both prescribed and non-prescribed – and the additional monitoring (physical and regulatory) that is required. The prescribing professional is often required to perform veritable 'juggling acts' to treat such complex conditions.

Neurological compromise may be the legacy of trauma while intoxicated or be a consequence of substance use-related violence. Additional causes may be a past history of acute cerebral hypoxia (low blood oxygen) due to high levels of brain depressant drugs (e.g. opioids or alcohol). In addition, brain injury may have occurred due to long-term use of alcohol (alcohol-related brain injury – ARBI).[12] All of these factors may impact on the person's thinking, reasoning and organisational processes, which may have implications for the way in which professionals are able to work with the affected individual.[12,13]

For those individuals who have active substance use problems, occurrence of withdrawal and intoxication may also complicate assessment of the individual as their terminal ill-health progresses. Ill-health related brain or hepatic deterioration may produce intoxication (including heavy sedation or coma) with substance use that was previously within the tolerance range of the individual. The interaction of increasing numbers of prescribed medications, including analgesics, increases the risk of interactions with alcohol and non-prescribed drugs. It is important to communicate these risks in a respectful non-judgemental manner to both the person receiving treatment and their family.

Sudden changes in presentation are of most concern. It is the family that are best placed to observe these changes on a day-to-day basis. Combinations of ill-health, significant medication interactions and psychoactive substances may lead to potentially fatal deteriorations. Non-judgemental conversations about past and ongoing substance use with the individual and family will help professionals to appropriately manage intoxication, withdrawal and potential deterioration.

Management of pain for the person experiencing palliation can be complex due to the myriad of psychological, biological and social circumstances often co-occurring in people experiencing substance use problems. Such complexities are not uncommon in the context of co-existing chronic pain disorders and long-term opioid use (prescribed and non-prescribed). Research has shown that opioid substitution treatment is associated with the development of a greater sensitivity to pain (hyperalgesia), regardless of opioid drug treatment for chronic pain or opioid addiction (slow-release morphine, methadone or buprenorphine).[14,15] Consequently, hyperalgesia, further development of pathology and significant pain tolerance to opioid analgesia may be observed in the palliative care setting, requiring major dose escalation. In contrast, sudden deterioration of organ function (particularly liver function) due to disease progression may result in rapid loss of tolerance and subsequent respiratory depression. This will necessitate re-assessment of currently prescribed medications, including those for the treatment of dependence and analgesia. A combination of dose reduction relative to change in tolerance and transfer to shorter-acting opioid agents (less problematic in terms of prolonged hepatic metabolism) should be considered. Reassurance should be given to the individual, as fear of pain and withdrawal are likely. Close monitoring will be required during this transition and a respite admission to a hospital or hospice palliative care setting would be appropriate.

PSYCHOLOGICAL CONSIDERATIONS

Mental health problems commonly co-exist with substance use problems.[16] Individuals who present to palliative care professionals may have a mental health diagnosis, including:

➤ substance use
➤ mood disorders
➤ anxiety
➤ psychosis
➤ personality syndromes.

All of these diagnoses have the potential to negatively affect the person's ability to cope with stressful situations. Importantly, the emotional stress provoked by the diagnosis of and suffering with terminal ill-health may affect the stability of the pre-existing mental health condition.

The 'self-medication' hypothesis for the development of substance use problems describes the individual's attempts to control depression, anxiety, post-traumatic stress disorder (PTSD) or psychotic disorders through the use of psychoactive drugs.[16] Conceptualising substance use in this manner helps the professional and the family both understand why the person receiving palliative care may increase their substance use.

The hazardous use of substances may be perceived as a maladaptive coping mechanism for life stressors. Many people experiencing substance use problems have experienced severe psychological stresses and social compromise. They are more likely to have experienced sexual or physical abuse, domestic violence, incarceration, and are more likely to be from socio-economically deprived backgrounds.[17] These negative experiences may exacerbate their end-of-life ill-health and present additional barriers to managing emotional, physical and spiritual aspects of the palliative care journey.

With any individual entering palliative care treatment, there may be a number of psychological 'mountains to climb', including grief and loss issues around identity as a worker, a partner, a parent or sibling. In addition, the loss of future roles as a grandparent or family elder may cause grief. For those experiencing substance use problems, the acceptance of these losses may be compounded by a sense of having lost years earlier in life to active substance dependence. For those who have made dramatic life changes in the hope they will enjoy a normal, happy life, these losses may create enormous psychological hurdles. There may be a sense of despair that these changes have not led to a more fulfilling life. Difficulty in negotiating these emotional 'minefields' may precipitate relapse to substance use, which may complicate delivery of palliative care options and result in unforeseen risks.

SOCIAL CONSIDERATIONS

Individuals who have had lives affected by substance use problems have frequently had difficulties in interpersonal relationships with their family, both pre-dating and subsequent to the development of their substance use problems.[16,18] The lifetime of challenges within these relationships and stress of the palliative diagnosis may complicate any simple resolution of problems during this period.

There may be a history of estrangement from the family of origin or from past partners, children and grandchildren. Past damage that has occurred both to the family and perhaps from the family, may be an issue the individual wishes to address at this seminal time. It is vitally important that they are well supported during this process. Reunion may be possible, although a large number of potential stressors may arise during this process. Importantly, exceptional levels of emotional stress may have significant impact on the experience of pain and use of substances during this time.[19,20]

For each individual the meaning of pain may be quite different (*see* Chapter 8). It is important to consider the effect of the development of chronic pain in terms of loss of employment and life roles, the effect on marriage and social interactions.[21]

RELATIONSHIPS

Identifying the level of support within family relationships is particularly important during the palliative care journey and this is no different for those experiencing substance use problems. It is known that having a supportive partner may reduce the emotional impact of pain. However, the expression of support by encouraging rest and decreased involvement with usual duties may contribute to the development of reported disability.[21] Regardless of age, it is also important to consider the impact of chronic pain on intimate relations between partners. Discussion of intimate relations with the individual may be uncomfortable for professionals and therefore it is often superficially addressed. However, such issues may be of paramount importance in relationships, no matter the age or level of disability. Experienced counsellors and psychologists are of great benefit to the person resolving issues with their partners while simultaneously contemplating other end-of-life considerations.

Indigenous issues

Relevant indigenous issues will vary depending on what part of the world the individual receiving care is in. It is important to ascertain the person's spiritual adherence to their cultural background as it cannot be assumed. Likewise, there may be socio-cultural beliefs that are not immediately obvious to the professional. Respectfully acknowledging the individual's beliefs and requesting further information as to the meaning of their cultural identity in the current circumstances is appropriate (*see* Chapter 4). It is possible that the person experiencing substance use problems may have become alienated from their socio-cultural group due to their substance use. The professional should encourage the individual to request support if he or she would like to address the issue.

CHALLENGES FOR PROFESSIONALS

The lack of experience or exposure to acute medical and psychiatric problems co-existing with substance use problems may provide considerable challenges for the palliative care professional when these concerns are compounded with end-of-life ill-health.

Concerns about misuse of prescribed medication may cause substantial uncertainty about what medications can or should be prescribed and what reasonable approaches can be used regarding dispensing instructions (*see* Chapter 8). Despite significant pharmaceutical company development, the production of opioid analgesia that is 100% tamper-resistant is not able to be guaranteed. Importantly, the professional should reflect on what concerns are realistic.

The reality of stigma attached to substance use problems, and those who experience them, cannot be denied. It is critical to understand the potential harms that may occur due to the clinical effects of this stigma. These harms may include underprescribing of analgesia despite our knowledge that opioid tolerance and hyperalgesia may warrant significant dose increments (*see* Chapters 7, 8). Additional harms may include discrimination towards the individual and their family. This may affect the engagement of the person with the team of professionals and their willingness to disclose pain, fears and unsanctioned substance use. It is important to note that older injecting drug users often experience more stigma and discrimination.[22]

A central issue that may arise due to stigma amongst substance users is incomplete disclosure to health professionals. Some people may feel that they will receive lesser quality healthcare if the professionals are aware of their substance use and may therefore withhold this information, potentially complicating healthcare planning and particularly pain management. Importantly, injecting drug users express concern that they will not receive adequate pain management if their identity as a past or present injector of drugs is revealed.[23]

In contrast, it is known that some controlled medicines prescribed to those receiving palliative care services will end up in the wrong hands.[24] It might be impossible to guarantee that this will not occur. However, some safeguards might be put in place. Limited dispensing to a carer may reduce the chance of diversion of medication. Good communication between hospital or hospice care professionals and community care professionals will help to monitor levels of sedation and/or drug effect in each setting. Any symptoms of sedation that the person reports may indicate lack of tolerance to the prescribed dose. These findings must be interpreted in the context of ill-health progression, which may also affect the tolerance at any given time. Baseline serum levels of opioids and/or benzodiazepines will give a useful comparison in cases of suspected medication diversion but also in cases of progressive organ deterioration affecting changes in tolerance. They can be used to guide reductions in dose alongside clinical observations as ill-health progression occurs.

Social circumstances of the affected individual may affect the setting in which care can be provided. In home situations where there is a known history of violence involving family or neighbours, safety assessments should take place and may involve seeing the person and the family at a community health setting. Other plans may be possible depending on the locality and on the outcome of the safety assessment.

Intermittent care provision in a community hospice or similar may be offered if there are few supports available in the home. This might provide respite for the family and may facilitate them to engage in any supportive therapy that might be indicated.

CONCLUSION

In conclusion, there is little reason to advocate for addressing substance use problems during palliative care unless this is requested by the individual. However, it is important to be aware of the many complexities of substance use problems and their potential effects on the needs of the individual and the family during end-of-life ill-health. The importance of respectful and ethical non-judgemental care delivered with unconditional positive regard is paramount (*see* Chapter 3). The duty of the professional is ultimately to provide factual information and support in a sensitive manner that respects the individual's right to make their own informed life choices while first doing no harm.

Case Study 14.1 – Josephine

Josephine (47) has been referred to palliative care services by a respiratory physician. She has end-stage chronic obstructive pulmonary disease (COPD) and has been on home oxygen for about 12 months. Her lung function has deteriorated considerably during this time and she is now essentially house-bound and is continually breathless at rest despite continuous oxygen.

She has been on daily methadone since the mid-1970s as a treatment for opioid dependence. She last used illicit drugs more than 10 years ago. Her partner is her carer and is also receiving daily methadone as a substitution treatment for past substance use.

Over the last eight months, Josephine has had a number of hospitalisations for management of deteriorating lung function. In addition, Josephine has had treatment for vertebral fractures associated with long-term high dose steroid treatment. Josephine also has chronic active hepatitis C, with the initial diagnosis of infection occurring about 20 years ago.

Increasingly, Josephine's presentations to the care team are associated with increasing pain and inability to tolerate this increasing pain. Her lung function continues to deteriorate and she remains hypoxic (low blood oxygen) despite continuous oxygen treatment.

When you attempt to talk to Josephine about possible changes in management she becomes angry and says, 'I'm dying, don't you know. I'm dying!'

SELF-ASSESSMENT EXERCISE 14.1 (*SEE* ANSWERS ON PP. 229–30)

Time: 45 minutes
- What are some of the challenges that might concern you?
- How might you prioritise monitoring and treatments?
- How might the professionals support the role of Josephine's partner?
- How might you respond to Josephine's anger?

REFERENCES

1 Cooper D. *Alcohol Home Detoxification and Assessment*. Oxfordshire/New York: Radcliffe Medical Press; 1994.
2 Winick C, Norman R. Epidemiology. In: Lowinson J, Ruiz P, Millman R, *et al.*, editors. *Substance Use: a comprehensive textbook*. 4th ed. Lippincott, Williams and Wilkins: Philadelphia; 2005.
3 Musto D. Historical perspectives in substance abuse. In: Lowinson J, Ruiz P, Millman R, *et al.*, editors. *Substance Use: a comprehensive textbook*. 4th ed. Lippincott, Williams and Wilkins: Philadelphia; 2005. p. 618.
4 Hojsted J, Sjogren P. Addiction to opioids in chronic pain patients: a literature review. *European Journal of Pain*. 2007; **11**: 490–518.
5 Dev R, Parsons HA, Palla S, *et al.* Undocumented alcoholism and its correlation with tobacco and illegal drug use in advanced cancer patients. *Cancer*. 2011; **117**: 4551–6.

6 Wolff AJ, O'Donnell AE. Pulmonary effects of illicit drug use. *Clinics in Chest Medicine*. 2004; **25**: 203–16.

7 O'Connor AD, Rusyniak DE, Bruno A. Cerebrovascular and cardiovascular complications of alcohol and sympathomimetic drug abuse. *Medical Clinics of North America*. 2005; **89**: 1343–58.

8 Darke S, Duflou J, Torok M. The comparative toxicology and major organ pathology of fatal methadone and heroin toxicity cases. *Drug and Alcohol Dependence*. 2010; **106**: 1–6.

9 Bhargava S, Arora RR. Cocaine and cardiovascular complications. *American Journal of Therapeutics*. 2011; **18**: e95–e100.

10 Karila L, Petit A, Lowenstein W, *et al*. Diagnosis and consequences of cocaine addiction. *Current Medicinal Chemistry*. 2012; **19**: 5612–8.

11 Megarbane B, Chevillard L. The large spectrum of pulmonary complications following illicit drug use: features and mechanisms. *Chemico-Biological Interactions*. 2013; **206**: 444–51.

12 Welch KA. Neurological complications of alcohol and misuse of drugs. *Practical Neurology*. 2011; **11**: 206–19.

13 Neiman J, Haapaniemi HM, Hillbom M. Neurological complications of drug abuse: pathophysiological mechanisms. *European Journal of Neurology*. 2000; **7**: 595–606.

14 Hay JL, White JM, Bochner F, *et al*. Hyperalgesia in opioid-managed chronic pain and opioid-dependent patients. *Journal of Pain*. 2009; **3**: 316–22.

15 Compton P, Canamar CP, Hillhouse M, *et al*. Hyperalgesia in heroin dependent patients and the effects of opioid substitution therapy. *Journal of Pain*. 2012; **13**: 401–9.

16 Allsop S. Introduction: mental health and drug problems: what is the issue? In: Allsop S, editor. *Drug Use and Mental Health*. Melbourne: IP Publishing; 2008. pp. 1–10.

17 Butcher J, Mineka S, Hooley J. Addiction disorders. In: Butcher J, Mineka S, Hooley J. *Abnormal Psychology*. 13th ed. London/New York: Pearson; 2007. pp. 421–6.

18 Baker A, Kay-Lambkin F. Co-existing mental health and drug and alcohol problems. In: Baker A, Velleman R, editors. *Clinical Handbook of Co-existing Mental Health and Drug and Alcohol Problems*. London/New York: Routledge; 2007. pp. 3–12.

19 Craig K. Emotions and psychobiology. In: McMahon S, Koltzenburg M, editors. *Wall and Melzack's Textbook of Pain*. London: Elsevier; 2006. p. 237.

20 Fields H, Basbaum A, Heinricher M. Central nervous system mechanisms of pain modulation. In: McMahon S, Koltzenburg M, editors. *Wall and Melzack's Textbook of Pain*. London: Elsevier; 2006. pp. 136–8.

21 Flor H, Turk D. Psychobiological mechanisms in chronic pain. In: Turk D. *Chronic Pain: an integrated biobehavioural approach*. Washington: IASP Press; 2011. pp. 89–136.

22 Anderson TL, Levy JA. Marginality among older injectors in today's illicit drug culture: assessing the impact of ageing. *Addiction*. 2003; **98**: 761–70.

23 Australian Injecting and Illicit Drug Users League (AIVL). *'Double Jeopardy': older injecting opioid users in Australia: AIVL Discussion Paper*. Canberra, Australia: Australian Injecting and Illicit Drug Users League; 2011.

24 Mercadante S, Craig D, Giarratano A. US Food and Drug Administration's Risk Evaluation and Mitigation Strategy for extended-release and long-acting opioids: pros and cons, and a European perspective. *Drugs*. 2012; **72**: 2327–32.

TO LEARN MORE

• Cooper DB, Cooper J, editors. *Palliative Care within Mental Health: principles and philosophy*. London/New York: Radcliffe Publishing; 2012.

• Hanks G, Cherny NI, Christakis NA, *et al*., editors. *Oxford Textbook of Palliative Medicine*. 4th ed. Oxford: Oxford University Press; 2010.

• Allsop S, editor. *Drug Use and Mental Health*. Melbourne: IP Publishing; 2008.

- Baker A, Velleman R, editors. *Clinical Handbook of Co-existing Mental Health and Drug and Alcohol Problems.* London/New York: Routledge; 2007.

ANSWERS TO SELF-ASSESSMENT EXERCISE 14.1 (*SEE* P. 227)

Challenges

- Quantifying pain and monitoring pain may be more difficult due to other co-existing ill-health. The prescriber of Josephine's daily methadone will be well placed to help to discriminate between discomfort associated with inadequacy or changes in the background methadone dose and pain from other origins. This might assist in developing a management plan for breakthrough pain (*see* Chapter 8) that is not controlled by regular doses of long-acting analgesia.
- Importantly, methadone treatment, when used as a substitution treatment for an opioid use problem, is sufficient to prevent withdrawal but is not a treatment for pain syndromes that present acutely or otherwise at a later date. In addition to this, analgesic requirements to treat pain may be substantially higher due to hyperalgesia and tolerance related to long-term opioid substitution treatment.
- Due to a long history of opioid dependence, the professional may experience concerns that there might be misuse of prescribed medications. There are a number of possible approaches to this situation, including more frequent dispensing of lesser amounts of medications and requesting that the person bring their medication for checking at clinic visits or when seen in the home by a professional. Openly acknowledging this concern at the outset while confirming a wish to work positively with the person is a useful way of providing the responsibility for safe keeping of medication to the person.
- There may be fears that the prescribed medication may interact significantly with the prescribed methadone, especially as there is progressive deterioration in organ function. Therapeutic serum drug levels may be a way of monitoring changes in medication metabolism (break down) as the ill-health progresses. This might allow for dose reductions at a later stage as appropriate. Open discussion of the potential for medication interactions and for tolerance to decrease causing increased sedation with Josephine and her partner will reduce the chance of distress if dose reductions are necessary at a later date.
- Legal prescribing requirements – these vary from jurisdiction to jurisdiction but certainly there are restrictions about prescribing drugs of dependence for individuals with known substance use problems. These can be clarified by contacting the prescribing department of your local health department, who may require a letter from a designated specialist confirming the person is now receiving palliative care from professionals. This will allow you to clarify ongoing legal requirements.
- It may be difficult for professionals to gain trust from Josephine and her partner if their past experience has been one of feeling stigmatised and discriminated against. Acknowledging that this may have occurred in the past might facilitate the development of trust and openness so that professionals can work more effectively with Josephine and her partner.

- There may be fears that Josephine's partner might misuse the prescribed opioid analgesia himself. He has a known history of opioid dependence and is prescribed methadone. He will need to be involved in the management of Josephine's medications and analgesia as her health deteriorates and her ability to access pharmacy services changes substantially. The degree to which this a logistical issue will change within the jurisdiction in which the prescriber is operating, and will need to be carefully monitored.

Monitoring and treatments
- Josephine might be reluctant to engage in conversation about potential changes in her regular medications in the event that the system is less able to cope and she demonstrates increased sedation. This might arise from an understandable fear that her pain may be inadequately managed. Close monitoring of pain and responsiveness to increases in pain might help to allay these fears.
- Close liaison with all professionals engaged in Josephine's care is essential.
- There may be a number of concerns and uncertainties regarding Josephine's partner. He may struggle to cope with the multiple demands involved in supporting Josephine while accessing care. Arranging support for him including some home help or similar would be of benefit. It is important to note that some people experiencing substance use problems who desperately need help will not seek or accept input due to past negative experiences including institutional discrimination.

CHAPTER 15

The heart of care and caring

David B Cooper, Jo Cooper

REFLECTIVE PRACTICE EXERCISE 15.1

Time: 60 minutes
- Now you have read this book, do you feel you have a better understanding of palliative practice within mental health in your work environment?
- *Think!* How can you apply this practice into your own area of care and practice?
- Who can you approach in order to instigate what you have learned into your own and others' practice?
- When will you do this?
- Make an action plan and deadlines for your actions and stick to them.

INTRODUCTION

The heart of caring is the knowledge and skill each professional holds and the humanity the professional shows to the person within their care. To ensure that professionals have the right level of skills and knowledge requires continuous training and supervision. This is not just for the student but for all professionals. It does not matter how much we feel we know, or how experienced we are, there is still the ongoing need to freshen up and learn new skills, developing new knowledge. It does not stop at a qualification.

The first step in disseminating knowledge and skill is a link person on each ward who is able to bring the skill and knowledge combining palliative care within mental health to the professional team. However, one 'specialist' professional on the ward is not enough. This professional's function is to bring the knowledge and skills of palliative care within mental health to all professionals working on the ward. The same approach applies in the community setting and care homes. Care needs to be taken when arranging professional updates or to improve the knowledge and skill sets in the 'student'. Each needs to be reassured that the 'mentor' is not suggesting a lack of skills or knowledge. Time should be taken exploring each professional's knowledge base and bringing these cohesively together to complement existing skills.

This is about taking the professional back to the roots of their knowledge base and drawing on each professional to examine and develop their understanding of palliative care within mental health – the heart of care and caring.

This requires a top down – manager to employees – and bottom up – employees to manager – approach to care and caring and to relearning that the professional is not just involved in high-tech care and targets but actual and active human-to-human contact, respecting each individual as unique in his or her own right.

It is acknowledged that test results, e.g. electrocardiogram (ECG), blood tests and so on, are important to that individual's care. However, whilst these results act as useful diagnostic tools they do not replace person-centred care – the human touch.

REFLECTIVE PRACTICE EXERCISE 15.2

> **Time: 30 minutes**
> Take time to reflect on your life and your place in the world, when you commenced your education and training. What did you hope to achieve for the person within your care? Now go back to that place.
> - Are you currently achieving these aims?
> - If not, why not?
> - How can you bring about the changes in your practice?
> - How can you share this new knowledge and skill with your fellow professionals?
> - What do you hope to achieve now?

TIME

We know that when asked about the care and caring side of practice and the ability to fully 'be with' a person – one human being to another – the immediate answer is 'we do not have time'! Yet it merely needs care and respect, showing the person that we care about his or her needs and want to help. A computer screen cannot do this.

It takes just one professional to care … a professional willing to plan and organise and make changes to current care and practice. For the manager, less time on paperwork and statistics, which encroach on the caring time, is everybody's responsibility. We can all act as agents for change.

SUPERVISION AND SUPPORT

The professional needs to self-confirm that supervision is not about the manager spying on the professional's practice. Moreover, to seek support is not a weakness but a willingness to learn and improve your professional human care and caring. How can we try to manage situations differently, producing a more desirable outcome for all concerned?

Clinical supervision and support is designed to help us to reflect deeply on the work we are doing, and how we do it. How it makes us feel and if our practice could be undertaken in a more meaningful and caring way. Perhaps 'supervision' should be renamed 'helpfulness programme'.

> Wisdom and compassion should become the dominating influences that
> guide our thoughts, our words, and our actions.[1]

Each of us, when undertaking this work, needs to acknowledge that we are all dependent on each other, whether we are junior or senior members of the care team. To
share such knowledge enables us to care and work with compassion (*see* Chapter 2).
However, it is not merely about being compassionate to others; we need to be compassionate to ourselves. If we are not, then we will fail to be compassionate to those
we care for and our fellow professionals.

WHAT WE HAVE LEARNED

As we have seen throughout these chapters, palliative care demonstrates many parallels with the care given in mental health practice. Therefore, it is not always obvious
– we just need to look for it when working on a busy ward, within the home and community or the care home environment to see that parallels exist. However, because of
their co-existence it should not be too difficult to adapt the processes, programmes
and aspects of care that run like a thread through many of these chapters. During all
your reflection on this book remember that it is just as important to look after yourself. This is something we often fail at, which can lead to a painful and distressing
personal and professional environment. Caring for ourselves needs inclusion in our
daily life and practice.

END OF CARING

It is a false belief that care and caring ends on discharge: our job is done and we can
move on to the next person. Care does not end when the person goes from our care.
The structure of continuing care and support needs to be meticulously planned before
we even think of discharge from our care.

   As with assessment, discharge should be planned early at the time of admission or
soon after, and should be ongoing. Care needs to be updated as the person progresses
from ill-health in our care to support and intervention or wellness at home. It is not
merely five minutes before 'chucking out time'.

MANAGING BEDS

It is not the practice professionals' task to manage beds. It has been observed by the
authors that the bed becomes more important than the individual within it ... we
are providing care and caring for a bed! People being discharged because there is a
need for a bed, regardless of their ability to be cared for at home or elsewhere – without consultation with the family – is ethically unsound and poor practice, still less
person-centred.

REFLECTIVE PRACTICE EXERCISE 15.3

Time: 30 minutes
- Consider the barriers for not instigating the palliative care approach.
- How do you feel you can overcome these barriers?
- Are the barriers real?
- Are they imagined?
- Either by yourself, or with a small group of colleagues, find a way to overcome any barriers and achieve a positive way forward.

IS IT ABOUT MONEY?

KEY POINT 15.1

With all the money in the world you cannot buy a caring, compassionate person or approach … this comes from within. It is not financial, it is about change in attitude towards care and practice by each professional.

COMMUNICATION

All the above is meaningless without effective communication between professionals and the person and family receiving compassionate care. What follows concentrates on effective communication, which is at the heart of care and caring.

KEY POINT 15.2

Effective communication is a master key … it fits all locks and opens all doors.[2]

SELF-ASSESSMENT EXERCISE 15.1

Time: 10 minutes
Consider the following
- When was the last time you wished communication within or outwith your team could be improved?
- What steps do you think you could take to improve the communication?

Effective communication can reduce the level of stress and burnout experienced by the professional. Sadly, burnout is no longer rare but an increasing level of risk for the professional in health and social care.[3]

Communication is pivotal when avoiding increased levels of stress and burnout. However, if this is the case – why do we often get it wrong? If effective communication is easy, why do we not practice it? If we are pleased when communication has gone well and angry when it has not, why do we have high expectations of others' effective communication and not pay attention to our own practices? If we are experiencing the effects of stress and burnout ourselves, why are we so unsympathetic to others when they experience the same?[3]

As individuals, we should know what to do and how to do it – there are no excuses. Yet we remain ineffective communicators, unless it impacts on us directly. Then we become experts – we notice how ineffective communication damages our day!

Here we provide a foundation for common courtesy and good practice that should be part of our professional and personal lives. We have become too familiar with poor communication and easily oversimplify or underestimate its importance. Consequently, we miss the value it holds for individuals, groups and ourselves.

WHAT IS EFFECTIVE COMMUNICATION?
Communication can be subdivided into seven parts:
1 individual, family and carers
2 junior team
3 peers
4 intra-disciplinary team
5 inter-disciplinary team
6 middle management
7 senior management.

Each is interdependent and interrelated – none stand alone.

> **KEY POINT 15.3**
>
> Integral to, and at the centre of all our actions, is effective communication with the individual, family and carers.[4]

Each person individually experiences the negative consequence of ineffective communication. Therefore effective communication is like the ripples in a pond, flowing effortlessly between each part.

Communication pond?
Water is made up of millions of individual molecules that collectively give water its fluidity.[4] Individuals within an organisation, or interlinked fields, are like the individual molecules of water. Each is interdependent on the other to provide the best possible quality of care for the individual, family and carers.

Imagine a stone landing in a pond. The ripples move seamlessly through the water until the pond is smooth, ready for the next stone. In this analogy, you are the stone – represented by *ME* in Figure 15.1. The *ME* is placed anywhere in the organisational structure. Wherever you are in the chart, *ME* is the centre for effective communication. It is your responsibility to ensure your communication flows effectively and effortlessly through the organisation.

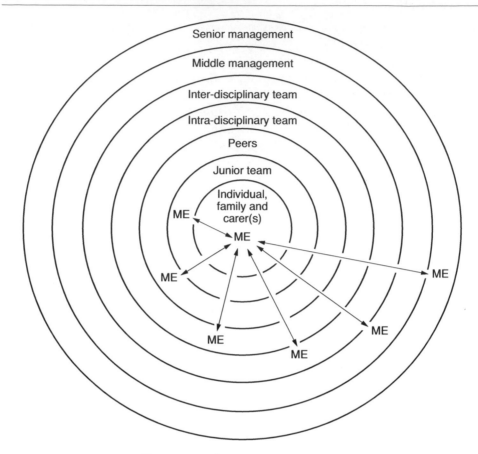

Figure 15.1 Communications pond

Effective communication therefore emanates like the ripples on a pond, flowing effort-lessly. Each professional having an equal responsibility to effectively communicate with the other, each intra- and inter-dependent. Only then can communication – and the care of the individual, family and carers – be effective.

1 Individual, family and carers

The individual, family and carers are central in any care environment. Every action, act or omission, from the junior member to the most senior manager, impacts on these individuals. Ineffective communication makes the treatment and intervention experience devastating and destructive.

The impact of verbal communication between professionals cannot be overemphasised.

How professionals share important and routine information related to the individual, family and carers does have a major impact on the successful outcome of any therapeutic intervention.[4]

With the individuals' permission, information relating to past and present health or social problems can be discussed with each professional or agency. Just as important is the information available from family and/or carers relating to the individual's concerns. The individual may forget or be unable to express important facts and information relevant to the presenting problem. Often, individuals and family can feel intimidated by the 'knowledgeable professional'.

The individual, family and carers can become dependent on the professional. This is not a deliberate act. It is easy to feel safe in the hands of a competent professional. The individual comes to depend on immediate access and consequently sudden unexpected and unplanned withdrawal is disruptive. The individual, family and carers should be informed at the outset about the level and extent of your involvement in their care. This should be periodically reinforced so the individual is aware of your end date.

Moreover, it is possible for the professional to extend contact with the individual, family and carers beyond that which is therapeutic. We gain subconscious reward from their dependence on us – the professional![4]

Careful monitoring and clinical supervision will aid awareness of such instances so that effective addressing of the negative aspects can be worked through ... and overcome.

Clinical supervision aids identification of overinvolvement and dependence, as well as exploration of our actions and omissions within care and caring.

Individuals do progress without our watchful eye if appropriate and effective intervention and treatment is managed effectively. We cannot protect them from all ills or dangers. Being aware of our limitations, intervention and the extent of the therapeutic value takes experience. Close monitoring of our actions is essential. A good indicator would be that when we come to write the legal records related to the individual and we have little to say about the person's progress, then it is time to evaluate one's effectiveness. Ineffective communication is damaging and destructive.

2 Junior team

Students and junior team members often feel isolated from the communication loop. Matters involving the organisation are heard on the grapevine, often half-factual, sometimes totally inaccurate.

> ### KEY POINT 15.6
> Effective communication with junior members of the team is just as important as in any other area of the organisation.

Unease and job dissatisfaction arise when the individual feels that he or she is unheard.

New employees are often unsure of the system and reluctant to express ideas and concepts for fear of reprimand or being labelled as troublemakers. Old hands do not always have the best or brightest concepts. Communication among and between junior team members and senior colleagues should be actively encouraged. Where possible, new ideas and initiatives should be given a fair hearing and encouraged. Yes, it may be that 'it has been tried before and failed', but maybe the time was not right or, indeed, the motivation. With supervision, support and encouragement, junior team members bring new ideas to the fore that can improve care, practice and communication.

Why is he or she doing this?

The easiest way to germinate suspicion and misunderstanding is to issue a directive that has no prior or present explanation as to its use. Suspicion can evolve to a negative response: 'Don't they think I am working hard enough?' 'Why are they watching me?' An explanation offsets the misconception, maintains productivity and improves working practice. Explanations of complex or role-changing information should be face-to-face. It is not acceptable to email or send a memorandum – this is at the least bad manners and certainly poor practice.

3 Peers

Communication upwards – managers are not clairvoyant – tell them!

A common complaint from team members is that the manager does not understand them. Like the manager, we, as individuals have a responsibility to communicate. Managers do not come to the post with a vacuum-packed crystal ball; nor are they clairvoyant – even if the issues seem blatantly obvious to you. Nor do they know everything there is to know about the workforce as a managerial tribal birthright. The manager needs clear and concise feedback. It is no use complaining that the manager does not appreciate the needs of your job, or that you are working in excess of your designated hours, if this is not explained to him or her. Likewise, it is no use complaining about the excessive workload and yet still working the excess hours for fear that this might jeopardise treatment, care and interventions: as professionals, we have a responsibility to communicate effectively too!

We cannot place all of the responsibility for ineffective communication on the manager! Each individual is capable of demonstrating how effective communication works. If we remain cognisant of the part each plays in ensuring that we are heard and understood, communication is effective and appreciation of each other's roles develops. In addition, each must exercise the ability to listen to others and analyse each individual's needs. Having listened, no effective change is achieved unless we act on the information and communicate it to others.

Peers are an effective means of support, supervision and guidance, yet we are often isolated in our professional practice. Stress and burnout causes ill-health.[3] We can all experience it. It is not a weakness.

KEY POINT 15.7

If we truly value one another, and wish to be effective in communication, and enjoy its rewards, we would be better placed to support, rather than dismiss, our colleagues. After all, it could be you next time!

---

4 Intra-disciplinary team
Communicating information
Some individuals within teams withhold information. To possess information not yet available to others is often misinterpreted as power. Practice and service provision is only effective if information is shared.

KEY POINT 15.8

There is more power and respect gained by sharing information and resources with colleagues than by withholding it.

After all, if no one knows you are holding that information – perhaps on a new treatment or approach – how can your influence and knowledge be acknowledged? Moreover, how can your colleagues improve treatment, care and interventions?

KEY POINT 15.9

Regular professional meetings are essential to information sharing.

If you are a hoarder by nature, this will be your opportunity to demonstrate your skill and knowledge, and at the same time bring the rest of the team up to date.

5 Inter-disciplinary team
The admission process
Whatever your area of work, the admission or acceptance of a planned therapeutic intervention with the individual, family and/or carers is part of your role. To be effective it is essential that professional communication is co-ordinated. Often the minor considerations have an important impact on ineffective communication if omitted.

In emergency hospital admissions, other hospital and community appointments can be missed. Other professionals and agencies involved may be unaware of the admission. Even planned admissions cause communication issues. Hospital admission provokes anxiety in even the calmest individual. People do forget to cancel appointments. Therefore, immediately the individual is engaged in assessment it should be ascertained what other services – directly or indirectly – are involved, and what appointments may be anticipated during admission. Planned appointments that may be missed, proposed community visits and/or clinic appointments need to be noted, and each professional colleague or agency should be informed. With permission, approach the family in case they hold additional information. In addition, direct communication with individuals and agencies by the professional is essential.

It is often easier to share information relating to your involvement with an individual using a multi-copy letter. It is good practice (and will be much appreciated by other colleagues) to give the individual a copy of this letter.

The discharge process

As the needs of the individual change, it may be appropriate to arrange a joint case/ family conference to share valuable information relating to the present and future care needs of the individual.

The individual, family and carers do feel vulnerable when intensive services are withdrawn. Even though the individual may require no immediate intervention, there is a sense of safety if it is understood that someone will be available to answer any questions they may have should a problem arise. Withdrawal of professional involvement or discharge should not take place until adequate arrangements for the continuation of essential care is agreed and in place. It is bad practice to withdraw a service or discharge the individual without adequate and effective planning. Crises can and do occur. Community services are not always easily accessible at weekends. Spending time on pre-withdrawal or discharge preparation will save one or more hours of crisis follow-up contact. Communication to the primary healthcare team is imperative to progress a smooth transition from hospital to home – even in rapid discharge.

KEY POINT 15.10

It is beneficial if the individual knows the name of the community or clinic professional who is involved in their follow-on care.

This is far more reassuring than being told that 'a letter will be sent to you in a week or so'. There appears to be an increasing delay when sending out discharge letters and/ or assessment letters. It is now common for such letters to take 3–5 weeks, and in some instances longer. Yet the person is given one week's supply of medication and/ or instructions to have sutures removed in 7–10 days. Such delay leaves the individual to act as go-between with the hospital/consultant and the general practitioner (GP)/ medical doctor (MD). Confusion can easily arise as the GP/MD does not always take on board what the person says in relation to medication or the feedback the person can give from their intervention or assessment.

> **KEY POINT 15.11**
>
> Common sense, courtesy and good manners form the basis of effective communication.[2]

6 Middle management
Communicating change

> **KEY POINT 15.12**
>
> The middle manager plays a pivotal role in the communication of change. Change in any organisation is unsettling.

Half-truth and rumours need little encouragement for dissemination and cause dissatisfaction. It is easier to have all your colleagues on board the ship than it is to stop the ship, circle and collect those who have fallen overboard. Change affects all members of the intra-disciplinary team; this in turn impacts on the inter-disciplinary team and ultimately individualised care and practice. To share, and be fully conversant with the change and the process involved, can and does lead to team support. Involvement and a sense of being part of the change process, rather than excluded and unworthy of consideration, are essential for effective communication and ownership of change.

An individual acting as a 'change agent' is beneficial ... but only if that professional has accurate information, has authority and standing within the organisation and manages his or her communications effectively. Effective communication is not about communicating with senior managers alone: it includes all professionals we work alongside, whatever the grade.

7 Senior management

Senior and middle managers need to know the detail of the job each employee undertakes. It is not essential for the manager to be from the same discipline, but it is necessary for him or her to be familiar with the exact role of the employee. Only then can respect, mutual understanding and communication be effective. Similarly, the manager needs to share with the employee what his or her own role entails.

Setting an example

During times of pressure and stress, effective communication is the first thing to suffer, yet it reduces pressure and stress. Effective communication frees time to deal with other matters that are important to individualised care. Effective communication comes from the top. Senior managers lead by example: only then will the employee find the tasks that he or she is set easier to work with and control. However, a lack of such leadership is not an excuse for one's actions, inactions or omissions.

The personal touch

Emails, texts and memos have made life easier for the busy manager. The increasing lack of pleasantries within the communication and the formal directness and abbreviation means that it is hard to perceive the literal intention of the message we receive. Managers should be aware of this change and make written communication accessible. Time to include the pleasantries should be spent when developing the communication. Avoid misinterpretation.

KEY POINT 15.13

Personal face-to-face communication is far more productive and fruitful in terms of manager and employee relationship.

It cannot be overemphasised that if the employee you wish to speak to is in the next room or same building and is immediately available, then stand up, walk out of the door and speak to him or her. This will be better received than an email or memo from someone who is only feet away. It establishes and earns respect.

TEAM TRUST

There is a need to seek and receive support and accept our own feelings. Being able to trust colleagues – be that a person of the same standing, junior or senior – and talk openly of our own feelings and experiences is essential.[5] Building trust is crucial to any team, and can only be achieved when each person feels a sense of security.

KEY POINT 15.14

Each individual has the right to be treated with respect, as intelligent, capable and equal human beings.

Eleven values of good quality teamwork[3,6]

1 **Humour** – There is a defined link between humour and good health, reduction of stress and creativity. Humour in the workplace:
   - improves productivity, person-centred services and morale
   - reduces sickness and stress
   - increases creativity
   - strengthens teamwork
   - enhances communication.[3,6]

   The power of humour:
   - teaches
   - inspires
   - motivates.[3,6]

Humour is effective as a:

> **best medicine** – laughing for the health of it
> **stress buster** – smiling to reduce stress
> **creative spark** – stimulates brain power
> **teaching aid** – use humour to reach your audience more effectively.[3,6]

However, there is a need to manage inappropriate humour by setting limits to what is not funny.

2 **Approachability** – It is important that colleagues feel another colleague is approachable. The freedom to discuss not only service and team development but concerns and problems, and openly ask for help, is essential.

3 **Identifying the needs of others** – Individually, team members need to be open-minded that others might not have the same expertise or coping skills. Offering help, guidance and support before it is requested is pivotal to skilled teamwork.

4 **Confidence and trust** – Confidence and trust is a hard-earned, but essential, individual characteristic of the successful team. All participants must embrace this team principle.

5 **Enjoyment of work** – It is 'okay' to enjoy your work, even when dealing with serious and enduring mental health problems, death and dying. There is much satisfaction in making someone more comfortable, or relieving physical, psychological, emotional and spiritual pain. Acknowledging that work is enjoyable, and sharing that with others, is okay.

6 **Practice sessions** – It is advantageous to hold formal practice meetings, at least monthly, where the team and professionals within the team can openly reflect on the quality of care and practice. The aim is to constructively develop good practice and to learn from experience without destructive criticism.

7 **Debriefing** – Whilst time-consuming, the benefits outweigh the few minutes spent ensuring that, at the start and end of each shift, each individual feels alright, and can freely discuss issues of concern, and not carry this home or into the workplace.

8 **Team building** – The annual 'awaydays' have a strong place in effective teamwork. The team meets, off-site, unencumbered by the workplace demands and expectations. The aim is to review how the team works together and how this could be improved and developed and to strengthen workplace relationships.

9 **Gossip and self-discipline** – It is destructive and bad practice for the team or individuals to talk about a colleague outwith his or her presence. This should not be encouraged or accepted. Each individual should hold his or her own court.

10 **Respect** – A feeling of team respect is essential. Each individual should feel valued and cared for. Sadly, whilst great emphasis is correctly placed on the value and care of the individual and family, we are often destructive in valuing and caring for our colleagues. Respect is earned by maintaining the values and practices outlined here.

11 **Time out** – No matter how dedicated one is, sometimes we need to take 10 minutes for ourselves during the working day. It permits the gathering of thoughts and emotions and/or putting into perspective something that has impinged upon

us during the shift. It clears one's head. Colleagues should expect, respect, accept and reciprocate this individual need. There should be no shame or guilt attached to taking 10 minutes to oneself.

CONCLUSION

A community psychiatric nurse in clinical supervision:

> Some managers feel that what we do is easy ... straightforward ... but it isn't easy and straightforward for the individual and family ... we have to help them untangle the web of dis-ease they find themselves facing ...[7]

This chapter reflects on a small number of examples of poor and ineffective communication and ways to improve communication, thus, reducing the level of stress and burnout[3] within our own work environment.

As we learn to look after ourselves we must not forget to learn to look after our colleagues, no matter what their role is within the organisation.

KEY POINT 15.15

It is about looking after each other and ourselves.

There is plethora of ineffective communication examples that one could describe: each one of us has our own personal story! This chapter aims to demonstrate that, with a little work from you, as an integral individual, effective communication leading to a good quality standard of care and caring can happen within and outwith your organisation: you just have to give it brain space and effort. It is not a thing to do later but an instrument to use constantly – always at the forefront of everyday activities.

Effective communication costs nothing. Misunderstanding, anger, frustration, complaints and worry – for the individual, family and carers, other professionals and oneself – can be avoided.

Having said all the above, none of this holds any importance if the receiver of communication does not listen. This two-way process is imperative if communication is to be effective.

No professional wants the individual, family or carers to suffer as a consequence of his or her inaction – yet we risk this every day through poor communication. It is not their responsibility – it is our responsibility to make communication effective and meaningful to the best of our ability and understanding. If there were just seven words of wisdom in professional practice and effective communication, these would be:

> ... never assume people know ... they do not![2]

The authors and editors hope that this book, and the preceding book (*Palliative Care within Mental Health: principles and philosophy*) have offered some insight into the application of introducing the practice of palliative care within mental health practice. The hope is that it has stimulated and motivated the reader on to good practice and further reading.

We have attempted to address the heart of care and caring throughout this book and hope that it may lead on to implementation. This chapter forms the final piece of effective and meaningful care and caring by addressing the importance of communication, which is placed as high in importance as any other care and practice covered in this book. Hopefully, this jigsaw is complete and we all can now progress to the heart of care and caring in our daily lives and practice.

> This tool, our body, is given to us for only a short time: this life.[8]

Let us use this tool to benefit the heart of care and caring.

REFERENCES

1 Matthieu Ricard. In: Föllmi D, Föllmi O. *Buddhist Offerings 365 Days*. London: Thames and Hudson; 2003. p. 30 November.
2 Cooper DB. Communication: the essence of good practice, management and leadership. In: Cooper DB. *Developing Services in Mental Health–Substance Use*. London: Radcliffe Publishing; 2011. pp. 161–70.
3 Davidson R. Stress issues in palliative care. In: Cooper J, editor. *Stepping into Palliative Care 1: relationships and responses*. 2nd ed. Oxford: Radcliffe Publishing; 2006. pp. 135–45.
4 Cooper DB. Looking after yourself and colleagues. In: Cooper DB, editor. *Palliative Care within Mental Health: principles and philosophy*. London/New York: Radcliffe Publishing; 2012. pp. 265–87.
5 Nichols K, Jenkinson J. *Leading a Support Group*. London: Chapman & Hall; 1991.
6 Fletcher-Cullum J. The value of teamwork. In: Cooper J, editor. *Stepping into Palliative Care 1: relationships and responses*. 2nd ed. Oxford: Radcliffe Publishing; 2006. pp. 129–31.
7 Anon – Community Psychiatric Nurse. 2012.
8 Dilgo Khyentse Rinpoche. In: Föllmi D, Föllmi O. *Buddhist Offerings 365 Days*. London: Thames and Hudson; 2003. p. 16 January.

TO LEARN MORE

• Cooper DB, Cooper J, editors. *Palliative Care within Mental Health: principles and philosophy*. London/New York: Radcliffe Publishing; 2012.
• Cooper J, editor. *Stepping into Palliative Care 1: relationships and responses*. 2nd ed. Oxford/Seattle: Radcliffe Publishing; 2006.
• Cooper J, editor. *Stepping into Palliative Care 2: care and practice*. 2nd ed. Oxford/Seattle: Radcliffe Publishing; 2006.

ACKNOWLEDGEMENT

The author is grateful to the editors and Radcliffe Publishing for permitting adaptation of this chapter:
• © In: Cooper J, editor. *Stepping into Palliative Care 1: relationships and responses*. 2nd ed. Oxford: Radcliffe Publishing; 2006. pp. 146–57.
• © In: Cooper DB, Cooper J, editors. *Palliative Care within Mental Health: principles and philosophy*. London/New York: Radcliffe Publishing; 2012. pp. 265–86.

Index

CPD with Radcliffe

You can now use a selection of our books to achieve CPD (Continuing Professional Development) points through directed reading.

We provide a free online form and downloadable certificate for your appraisal portfolio. Look for the CPD logo and register with us at: www.radcliffehealth.com/cpd

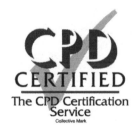